Get Your Life Back

Get Your Life Back

A Step-by-Step Recovery Guide for

Chronic Fatigue Syndrome

Toby Morrison

Myalgic Encephalomyelitis—also known as ME/
CFS or chronic fatigue syndrome—will be referred to as
CFS throughout this book for ease of reading.

First published in 2026 by Dean Publishing
PO Box 119
Mt. Macedon, Victoria, 3441
Australia
deanpublishing.com

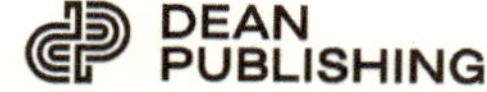

Cataloguing-in-Publication Data
National Library of Australia
Title: Get Your Life Back
ISBN: 978-0-648938-66-8
Category: Personal health/chronic fatigue syndrome

The views and opinions expressed in this book are those of the author and
do not necessarily reflect the official policy or position of any other agency,
publisher, organization, employer, medical body, psychological body, or
company. Assumptions made in the analysis are not reflective of the position
of any entity other than the author(s)—and, these views are always subject to
change, revision, and rethinking at any time.

The author, publisher or organizations are not to be held responsible for
misuse, reuse, recycled and cited and/or uncited copies of content within
this book by others.

The ideas within this book are based on the author's experience and are not
intended to replace any professional advice or diagnose or treat any health
or mental issues. This book is not intended to treat health or psychological
issues but act as a reflective and inspiring resource for personal health.
Chronic fatigue syndrome is a multi-faceted subject with differing opinions
and recommendations, the reader is advised to always seek professional
advice according to their specific needs.

The stories and ideas in this book stem from the author's experiences and
are created from memory. Some names and identifying details of others
have been changed to protect the privacy of individuals.

FREEDOM begins here

You're not crazy.

You're not lazy.

You're not alone.

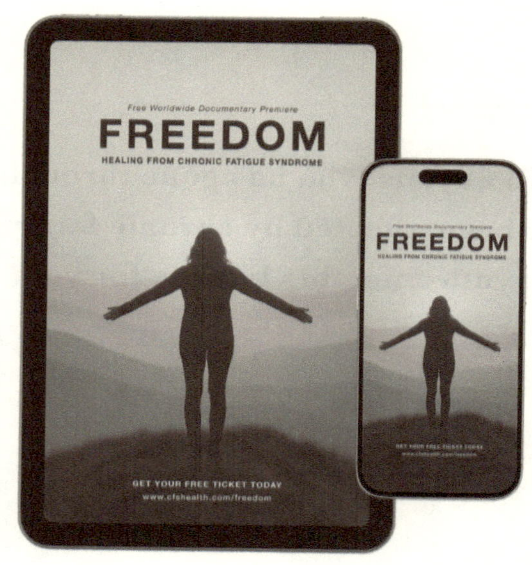

Free Worldwide Documentary

www.cfshealth.com/freedom

CONTENTS

PREFACE

Since my first book on chronic fatigue syndrome twelve years ago, my philosophy on treating chronic fatigue syndrome has evolved. Within the fifteen years of helping thousands of clients recover, I have developed a more comprehensive strategy with specific steps for the recovery process to happen.

What I share in this book has helped thousands of people in 78 countries get their lives back; it's my hope that this book helps you do the same.

I had chronic fatigue syndrome twenty years ago, and it was one of the hardest, most excruciating, painful periods of my life. I promised myself that when I got better, I would make sure no one else had to suffer like I did. I have kept that promise, and it has been the catalyst for creating CFS Health—helping thousands through our online recovery program, producing a documentary, launching a podcast and YouTube channel, and ultimately writing this second book, *Get Your Life Back.*

Throughout this book you will read incredible stories of real people just like you who completely turned their health and life around. People who once felt helpless, lost, and devastated by this crippling syndrome.

What you are going through is very real. It's very hard. But recovery is possible.

CFS Health doesn't stand for chronic fatigue syndrome, it stands for **C**hoice, **F**reedom, **S**uccess. And I believe that people who refuse to give up deserve to start living again. The fact you have this book in your hand shows me that YOU are someone who doesn't give up.

In the inspiring words of Janet Crabbie, our eldest CFS member who recovered at age 86: **"Don't give up, as tomorrow is a chance for better days."**

If you're suffering from chronic fatigue syndrome, I have good news and bad news. The bad news is that those who haven't experienced CFS are unlikely to fully understand how you feel so it can be lonely and isolating. The good news is that you don't need everyone to fully understand you or CFS for you to get better. What's even better is this: it is possible to get your life back. And that's what this book is all about—*you and your life*.

Let's begin.

CHAPTER 1

It's Not Your Fault

The room was pitch black. I lay in bed, in total agony from head to toe. My muscles felt like lead and a fire raged inside my body. Exhausted, defeated, and ready to give up, my father entered my room.

I stared at him, almost paralyzed from pain. A far cry from where I was years prior—a fit, healthy, young man in my prime.

"Why me, Dad?" I asked, barely managing a whisper.

He sat next to me and placed a gentle but comforting hand on my leg.

"I don't know why right now, son, but what I do know is one day you will look back at all this and be thankful for it; you'll realize it was for a bigger reason."

Dad was a gentle and wise man by nature, but this time his "wisdom" did not penetrate. My mind spun. My nervous system flared. *What? How could I be thankful for this?* I wanted to slap him for even saying that! *Was he being cruel? What did he mean by that? Was he right?*

I didn't know what he meant by "a bigger reason" all those years ago. But I do now. *(It turns out he is pretty wise after all)*.

Imagine this…you guzzle twenty alcoholic drinks, then run a marathon, then take a twenty-hour flight…you suffer horrendous jet lag, and don't sleep for three days straight. Then, on top of that, you get flu symptoms-razor-blade throat, acute headaches, chronic muscle aches, body pain, swollen lymph nodes and brain fog so bad you forget what you said a minute ago.

Well…that's what it's like to have chronic fatigue syndrome. And it's real.

And…it's **NOT. YOUR. FAULT.**

If you're suffering with CFS right now, you've probably been told by doctors or friends things like:

"You just need to think positive."

"Maybe you're depressed."

"It's all in your head."

"Everyone's tired, get on with it."

"Sweat it out."

And…"There's nothing you can do about it."

Perhaps you have well-meaning friends and family who send you website links to supplements or wacky gadgets that "will apparently 'cure' chronic fatigue syndrome." Or they tell you that there's a person down the road who treats people with chronic fatigue syndrome, and "you should give it a try."

They mean well, but it doesn't help.

You feel stuck with chronic fatigue syndrome, and it sucks, bad. It's so bad, you wouldn't wish it upon your worst enemy.

And one of the hardest parts is that it's often dismissed as something psychological—"all in your head."

In the 80s, when the illness was beginning to be recognized, some media commentators termed it the "Yuppie Flu"; a derogatory name implying that this debilitating syndrome is nothing more than hypochondria, or a case of burnout. *Gee, thanks.*

If you have chronic fatigue syndrome, you know the symptoms are hardcore.

You know the deal:

- pain in the joints or muscles
- whole body fatigue
- an inability to exercise
- cognitive confusion
- forgetfulness and difficulty with concentration
- excessive sleepiness or sleep disturbances
- headaches and sore throat
- swollen glands and malaise
- muscle weakness
- sensitivity to pain
- brain fog
- dizziness
- noise and light sensitivity
- post-exertional malaise (PEM)

Millions of people worldwide suffer from chronic fatigue syndrome (CFS) or myalgic encephalomyelitis (ME) as it's also known. It's estimated that around 5% of the population suffer, and it's linked to a multitude of factors including a virus like glandular fever or COVID-19.[1] Recent studies have shown there could also be links to genetics and an alteration in the immune system.[2]

Despite this knowledge, there is no hard-and-fast cause, no easy way to get diagnosed, no official treatment plans, and most damaging of all, no "cure."

In fact, estimates indicate that up to 90% of people with CFS/ME may be undiagnosed.[3] The small percentage of people who do get diagnosed are often told there's nothing they can do but to rest and try to get on with their lives. To me, that's NOT a solution.

CFS also often comes with fibromyalgia—a disorder characterized by widespread musculoskeletal pain, and fatigue, sleep, memory and mood issues. Researchers believe fibromyalgia amplifies painful sensations and affects the way your brain and spinal cord processes painful and non-painful signals. The percentage of overlap between fibromyalgia and chronic fatigue syndrome is estimated to be quite high, with one study showing that 58% of fibromyalgia cases met the full criteria for CFS.[4]

And if that's not enough to contend with, on top of those primary symptoms comes the secondary suffering—sadness, frustration, guilt, shame, isolation, anxiety, depression and a sense of malaise. Not to mention the interpersonal challenges, loss of identity, and crippling lack of social life.

It is debilitating.

And…**YOU. ARE. NOT. ALONE.**

**To understand fatigue in chronic illness,
a healthy person would need to stay
awake for three days straight...and
then try to function like normal.**

Understanding chronic fatigue syndrome is vital because with understanding comes awareness. Here are eight important facts about CFS everyone needs to know:

1. Chronic fatigue syndrome can feel like an invisible illness. People may not understand your struggles, which can be really frustrating.

2. Losing friends when you have chronic fatigue syndrome can happen, and it is painful. It can be hard to find new connections who understand what you're going through.

3. Family members can feel a sense of loss when you're dealing with chronic fatigue syndrome. They want you to get better, but the pressure can be overwhelming.

4. The guilt that comes with chronic fatigue syndrome can be crushing. You don't want to disappoint your friends and family, but you also need to take care of yourself.

5. Suffering from chronic fatigue syndrome can lead to secondary emotions like guilt and sadness. It's important to acknowledge these feelings and work on letting them go.

6. Finding a supportive doctor who understands chronic fatigue syndrome can be challenging. It's important

to keep advocating for yourself and seeking out the right support.

7. Chronic fatigue syndrome is not just feeling tired all the time. It's a complex illness that can impact every aspect of your life, from work to relationships and hobbies.

8. Going through chronic fatigue syndrome is a daily battle, but you are not alone. There is support out there, and there are ways to improve the quality of life and wellbeing.

NOW IMAGINE THIS...

Most people who never go through CFS just think it's a psychological problem. Until I ask them to imagine their life full of fun and activity. For example, let's say you love bike riding, you love your job, and meeting up with friends and family. Let's say you usually wake up at 6am and go for a one-hour bike ride before work. You have breakfast, get changed, go to work, do a full day, go out for dinner with friends, have a late night, and do it all over again the next day. Totally fine. No issues at all. Life is good.

Until the very next day...when the carpet is swept from beneath your feet. You can barely get out of bed. You struggle to get to the bathroom, your day consists of bed, rest, food, sleep—repeat. You're in constant pain, and talking for more than five minutes is exhausting.

Your life went from hero to zero real quick. Without warning, without consent. A complete blindside. Yep, this is chronic fatigue syndrome. It doesn't play fair. In fact, it hardly lets you play at all.

The uncertainty that accompanies chronic fatigue syndrome in the beginning is super tough. You can be struck with a variety of different symptoms that could be anything. Not knowing is scary and frustrating. The intensity of symptoms and unanswerable questions causes further energy depletion.

Then comes the isolation that comes with feeling chronically unwell, and this magnifies the discomfort in your mind. It can become a vicious loop of worry and despair.

You shut yourself off from the world, go into your bedroom, and rest all day. You do nothing out of a fear of doing too much, or doing the wrong thing, which creates more uncertainty, which keeps you trapped. Dr. Google becomes your best friend and your worst nightmare.

The myriad of overwhelming information available at your fingertips compounds the confusion. You wonder: *What do I do? Do I focus on my diet? Do I focus on not exercising? Do I focus on exercising? Do I get a coach? Do I join this program or that one? Do I take this supplement? Or try this new pill or potion?*

There's a lot of free information out there, which is great, but it can be all too much. *Analysis paralysis*—the state of overthinking a decision to the point where making any choice feels impossible—can set in big time. And you can barely function, let alone take some kind of action.

Sound familiar? Yup, it's A LOT!

Having chronic fatigue syndrome is like trying to live your life underwater—every movement takes ten times the effort.

But today, things change.

I know how tough this syndrome is because it forced its way into my life when I was sixteen. For the next four grueling years I was bedridden with severe symptoms. But now I am fully recovered. Not only have I gotten my life back but so have thousands of other people like me.

A lot of medical people pedal the belief that you can't get better with chronic fatigue syndrome. But…THAT IS NOT TRUE.

People are getting better **ALL. THE. TIME.**

In our program, people are working, hiking, parenting and exercising. Annabel has been on a four-month holiday, Claire has just started full-time work, Carly just got married. And Mary has become a grandmother; and loving every moment of it. Blake swims two kilometers in the ocean most mornings for fun (which is a far cry from where he was bedbound ten years ago). Just the other day I received a message from a past client, Beth, telling me she just gave birth to her daughter. Pretty amazing considering ALL these people were either told there is nothing they could do, or at one point they didn't believe recovery was possible for them.

The crazy thing is these stories sound almost too good to be true, but if you saw them at their worst, you would barely recognize them today.

Recovery certainly didn't happen overnight for these folks. It happened over time. But as you will learn through this book, **doing the right things at the right time, gets the right results.**

It is entirely possible; in fact, it happens often.

Believing the myth—"there is nothing I can do'"—can create "illness identity" (the degree to which an illness is incorporated into one's identity) and this identity can keep you stuck in CFS for longer than you need.

Here's the thing. Let me say it again—*It's not your fault.* Chances are you've been told your situation is helpless, that you must "deal with it" for the rest of your life. If this is you, please stop beating yourself up. What you're going through is hard enough. You don't need additional layers of pain.

But from today on, things change. *There is another way.*

There is hope.

THE TWO WAYS OF LOOKING AT IT

In my opinion, there are two ways of looking at this illness.

The first way is to believe there is nothing you can do and hold the fixed belief that you just have to "live with it." How would life feel if you had to live with this debilitating condition for the rest of your life? It would be heavy and hard. You can understand why so many sufferers battle with depression and anxiety if they're told there's no end in sight.

The second way is to know that recovery is possible. Why? Because you know for a fact that people get better. You've seen it online (watch CFS Health Success Stories on my YouTube channel to see what I am talking about) and you'll see it throughout this book.

The first way keeps you right where you are stuck.

The second gives you possibilities.

If you choose the second way and believe that recovery is possible, you can then begin to take a proactive approach towards your recovery. And that is a game-changer!

At the end of the day, you have to get into the driver's seat of recovery. If you are looking for external things outside of you to "fix you" then getting better is always elusive. I haven't seen it in fifteen years of working with clients. But if you take the driver's seat and follow the right pathway and process, you will discover that recovery is possible, and so is getting your life back.

And that's what this book is all about.

You see, I've noticed something fascinating about those who recover. They all seem to have six major things in common. Spoiler alert: I'm about to spill the beans…

1. They realized it was possible to get better.
2. They stopped trying quick-fix after quick-fix after quick-fix (it ain't so quick).
3. They took a holistic approach. It was never just one thing that got them better, it was always a multitude of processes done at the right time, over time.

4. They stay committed to the recovery. Not just a 3/10 commitment, but a full-blown 10/10.

5. They didn't measure time or constantly ask, "How long is this going to take?" (Ticking time bomb mentality doesn't work. You are already under enough pressure, adding time pressure is a sure way to stunt progress.)

6. They participated in their recovery and took full responsibility in making changes.

And here's the kicker—*you* **can be one of these people.**

That's right. **Your diagnosis doesn't have to be your final destination.**

How would you feel if you could build a new life not riddled with symptoms and struggle? Well…I'm here to tell you, you can. That's the reason I formed CFS Health, created a documentary, and wrote this book. *You* **are the reason.**

You see, I didn't want anyone to endure the unnecessary suffering and isolation that I experienced over twenty years ago. Like many, I tried every miracle gadget and bizarre therapy I could find. Some offered mild relief, but none provided the answers. So I became the answer. And although it was a windy road to recovery, I did fully recover. I also found out that the way to recovery wasn't found in the latest high-tech health devices with outlandish names all promising to make my symptoms vanish. It wasn't found in glossy marketing remedies or "overnight" success stories. It was built through trial and error with a holistic approach in mind. In the following chapters, I break down the same process thousands of others from all over the world have used to reach recovery and live their lives again.

But before we do that, we need to talk about the biggest initial recovery blocker I see people go through—acceptance.

Now, when I say *acceptance,* I don't mean resignation, nor do I mean to shrug your shoulders and just say, "oh well, that's it, there's nothing I can do." I truly mean that the first step to recovery lies hidden in acceptance.

Let me explain...

ACCEPTANCE IS THE FIRST STEP TO RECOVERY

Why is acceptance so vital? Here's what I have come to know. What we resist persists. What we reject, we don't accept.

And what we don't accept we cannot change.

One of the hardest parts about CFS is acceptance. The loss of identity is brutal. I am sure CFS was not in your plans, or goals of life.

When I battled CFS, I was angry with the world. I was so upset that I couldn't do the things that made me, *me.* My whole world turned upside down, and there were nights I would cry myself to sleep asking, *Why me? WHY MEEEE?*

It felt unfair. Like I didn't deserve it, I didn't do anything wrong to deserve CFS in my life. And, I'm sure you didn't ask for this situation either. But here you are. It sucks. It can feel like you're in a constant tug-of-war with yourself. Constantly comparing yourself to all your friends and peers. Constantly comparing your current life with your old life. Your old energy levels to your current ones.

The hurt is real. The guilt is real.

BUT…it wasn't until I accepted my current reality that I could actually change it.

Many people fear that accepting their condition means they've failed, that they're giving up, that they're beaten. But that is not the truth.

It's normal to resist accepting your current reality, especially when it's so far from what you wanted or expected. The life you knew before CFS, or any other serious illness, feels worlds away. But let me be clear: acceptance doesn't happen overnight, and it certainly isn't easy. There is no quick fix, no magic cure. However, when you begin to consistently do the right things at the right time, progress happens. And it's incredible.

It's perfectly okay to feel the heavy burden that comes with CFS—grief, guilt, and a sense of resignation. This emotional weight is heavy. But acceptance, when understood correctly, is not resignation.

Let me share something I said to a client Mark during one of our weekly Q&A sessions. Mark was struggling with anger and frustration; he found it very difficult to accept his illness. He was petrified to accept his current situation because he believed that meant he was giving up or being complacent and would never get better as a result.

I said to Mark, "I know it's scary, but once we accept your current situation, you can change it, until that happens, nothing will change for the better. It can feel like you're living in quicksand, and no matter how hard you try, you keep sinking lower and lower each time."

He nodded. He knew all about that sinking feeling. He knew all about trying too hard.

I asked Mark. "What if acceptance is the starting point to getting better?"

Mark sighed. "I guess it's worth a try then."

I reassured him that I wasn't asking him to "give up." I was inviting him to give up his resistance.

Imagine if we viewed acceptance as a starting point. This tiny shift in perspective changes everything. Without acceptance, we're stuck in a loop of frustration, asking "Why me?" and believing that life is unfair.

**Acceptance doesn't mean you agree with
or even like your current situation.
It means you acknowledge it as your reality
so you can start to move forward.**

You accept that this is not the end—but the beginning of your journey. When you embrace this mindset, the path ahead starts to look a lot more like a stairway of progress, rather than a downward spiral, **because accepting where you are at means you can START where you are with your recovery.**

Acceptance allows you to see things as they are and focus on what you can do, rather than what you can't do.

A mindset of proactive acceptance acknowledges the situation without succumbing to it. This approach was the catalyst for my recovery, and ultimately it will be the starting point for change for you too. Yes, proactive acceptance is the first key to a new life heading towards 'destination recovery'.

Calmness *with* acceptance

Acceptance enables a clear perception of reality, allowing the situation to be seen with logic and practicality. In our program, acceptance *with calmness* is vital. We don't allow people to do our programs in a desperate state of mind. Why? Because you won't get better. Why? **Because you can't recover from the same state you got sick in.**

Read that again. *You can't recover from the same state you got sick in.*

It's not your fault but it is a fact.

Recovery works when it comes from a place of calm acceptance and practicality. When you're at ease and doing the right things at the right time, you'll notice an upward progression in your health—better sleep, improved digestion, and a calmer nervous system. You start to feel better because you're reconditioning your body appropriately. Calmness settles down the nervous system and from there, healing happens.

Once you embrace the idea that acceptance is a starting point, things can change rapidly. We've seen it time and again with our members. It's only from ease that you can create nourishing daily habits without pressure.

Ask yourself this:

- *How would it feel to simply accept "what is" and start to recover?*
- *How would it feel to stop self-rejection and begin a pathway of self-love and compassion?*

Acceptance is the foundation upon which you can build the life you want, not the life you've lost.

You can stop blaming yourself. It's not your fault. The system has let you down and you've most likely been left in the medical desert not knowing what to do. So do not beat yourself up for where you are right now. Stop comparing yourself now to your old self. I know it's hard, but what you are going through is hard enough. Take some pressure off.

It's my belief that **recovery is hard, but *not* recovering is harder.**

Recovery isn't about trying to get back your old life, it's about building your new life.

TAKEAWAYS

CFS is an invisible illness characterized by severe fatigue, cognitive issues, and physical pain, often leading to isolation and misunderstanding from others.

Sufferers experience secondary emotional challenges, including guilt, sadness, anxiety, and frustration, compounded by the loss of their former active lives.

Acceptance as a starting point and is essential for recovery. Acceptance is not resignation but the foundation for taking proactive steps towards improvement.

A calm, accepting mindset is crucial for recovery. Stress and desperation can hinder progress, while calmness enables the body to heal more effectively.

Recovery is possible through a holistic, multifaceted approach, focusing on consistent, appropriate actions over time rather than quick fixes.

RECOVERY INSPIRATION

Get inspired by people just like you who have overcome CFS—download our free compilation of case studies now.

CHAPTER 2

The Fight of My Life

Growing up, I was known as the kid who was always on the go. I was full of energy: nothing could hold me back. When my mom was pregnant with me, she said she'd never had so much energy in her life; she would walk twenty kilometers a day, which strangely she had never done until she was pregnant with me.

In my early teens, sport was my life. I was an elite basketball player and had played at a high level from the age of twelve. By the time I was sixteen, I was playing in three different teams, trained five nights a week and played three games a week. I was also representing my school in athletics and team sports and doing extra gym sessions when I could. I was completely sports mad.

At the time, I didn't give any thought to how much exercise I was doing, and I was oblivious to the strain I was putting on my body and mind. The philosophy back then was "no pain, no gain" and so I pushed hard all the time. It was all or nothing.

Then one day I came down with glandular fever, also known as "mono," and my body went into meltdown. I thought it was a normal cold and flu and I would get over it in a few days. I had no energy and there were days where I couldn't lift my head off the pillow. I was seriously sick and there was nothing I could do about it. The doctors told me to rest and said I would be fine in a month or two. But I wasn't.

No matter how much I rested, my symptoms only got worse. **If rest cured fatigue, I'd be healed by now.**

I suffered extreme lethargy and fatigue, brain fog, swollen glands, sore throat, achy legs, dizziness and gut problems. My sleep was affected by these symptoms, and I developed insomnia and restlessness as well. For nine straight months, I had no idea what was wrong with me. My life shrank so rapidly from bubbly and energized to weak and exhausted. It was an extremely scary time, and because of the uncertainty and such ill health, I thought I had cancer.

After nine months of seeing specialist after specialist, being tested for every illness under the sun and having what felt like hundreds of blood tests, I was finally diagnosed with chronic fatigue syndrome.

In that moment of diagnosis, I was relieved. I thought I finally had an answer. But by the time I left the doctor's office, I felt sick in my stomach and totally deflated because he told me there was nothing I could do to get better.

"You have to rest and wait and see," he said.

I remember that night vividly. I came home in total rage. I felt so stuck. It was supposed to be a day of happiness and relief, but without an answer of what to do, I felt overwhelmed.

The diagnosis felt like a life sentence. That there was no way I would be able to get my life back and that my life would suck forever.

**It never occurred to me that one day,
I'd wake up sick and not get better.**

I paced to my bedroom, picked up a basketball shoe I hadn't worn in over nine months and threw it as hard as I could at my bedroom wall and screamed! As the shoe dropped, I fell to the ground and sobbed. Tears streamed down my face like a waterfall. Defeat consumed me.

I cried myself to sleep that night, praying that I would wake up and things would be different. But when I woke, *everything* was the same.

THE INVISIBLE BATTLEGROUND

Three long years went by.

I missed most of my senior school years, my teenage social life, and many family events. My sports activities came to a complete stop. I felt as though I had no life left. I had gone from being a social butterfly and a super fit sports fanatic to bedbound and struggling to lift my head off the pillow. My dream to become a famous basketball player in America was gone. The only dream I had left, was if I were to get better one day, then I would make sure that no one else would suffer alone like I did.

During the four years I battled chronic fatigue syndrome, I was told countless times that the illness was all in my head. Teachers and other people in my life would say that I was making it up. Some even accused me of being lazy and a "bad student." That I needed to "think more positively" and "sweat it out" or that I was "just depressed."

It's hard being someone who wants to do everything, stuck in a body that struggles to do anything.

I was told so many times that there was nothing that could be done. It made it extremely hard to stay hopeful.

For a long time, I did not believe that recovery was possible. I saw the rest of my life as an existence of pain and misery. There were days when I didn't want to wake up and days I wished my life was completely over because the suffering and pain was so immense. I even once told Mom that I didn't feel like being here anymore. We both cried. The illness was taking everything from me, even my sense of hope.

There were many reasons why I wanted to give up, but I want to share one that hits really deep: the reason I wanted to give up was because I didn't want to let go of my old life. It affected me so much that it delayed my recovery by years. I was tied to a sense of identity and fixated by the fact that I couldn't be 'that person' anymore. The loss of my 'old self' created deep pain and suffering for me.

Chronic illness isn't just physical pain; it's canceling dreams for doctor visits, feeling your body betray you, and hearing,"but you don't look sick."

The other thing that cut deep was that I was exiled from my friendship group. One day you've got friends, then, all of a sudden, you're the odd one out. I got bombarded with questions: "Why aren't you at school?" "Why aren't you playing sport?" "Why can't you come to the movies?"

I didn't know what was wrong with me, so I couldn't even explain myself properly, let alone to others. There was this constant back and forth with friends and misunderstandings and hurtful comments, with people saying that I was making it up, that I was just depressed (I was depressed but that was a symptom of the cause, not the cause of the symptoms), or I needed to be more motivated.

How could I explain the unexplainable? Like the fact…

- I cancel plans I desperately want to attend.
- I rest for hours after a shower.
- I forget basic words mid-sentence.
- I grieve a version of myself I barely remember.
- I fight every day for a body that doesn't cooperate.
- That I'm not just tired. I'm chronically ill, and no one understands.
- That I'm not lazy, I'm just fighting a battle you can't see.

Sound familiar?

The truth is I deeply missed my old life. I missed myself. I missed who I was. I missed the version of me that didn't have to think about my energy levels before doing something. I missed being understood. I missed my friendship circle. I missed sports. I missed happiness.

My life and my identity had been dismantled, and I was left with only rubble.

For people with CFS this is reality. And the truth is that no one, not even family members and close friends, can fully understand what you are feeling and experiencing.

It's not that you don't want to do things; it's that your body won't let you, right?

You see, there are some things that only people with CFS understand about CFS. And it's not that you don't want to explain them, it's just that you're too tired to fully explain them. Things like:

I'm not lazy; I'm exhausted.

I cancel plans because I have to, not because I want to.

Rest isn't a luxury; it's a survival strategy.

I'm grieving the life I used to have.

Being told to "just push through" makes it worse.

I want to feel better more than anyone else.

It's like trying to explain an invisible battleground with an invisible 'enemy' and you're the prey. Others can't see it fully, but you face the battle every-single-day.

The years spent battling chronic fatigue syndrome were some of the hardest times of my life. One of the things that helped me get through those dark times was that I held on to a better future. **It was only when I accepted my current reality that I allowed myself to move forward.**

Accepting who I was *now*, helped me finally realize that recovery isn't about trying to get back your old life, it's about building your new life. It's about getting your life back in a new way.

TURNING POINTS

This revelation of radical acceptance helped a lot, but I still wasn't fully equipped with everything I needed to start my recovery.

By this point, I had seen all types of specialists from all different medical backgrounds, and it hadn't helped much at all. I had tried almost everything: physios, nutritionists, naturopaths, psychologists, gut specialists, Chinese medicine, supplementation, acupuncture, chiropractors, and weird whacky doctors. You name it, I tried it. Some of it helped a little, but nothing made a difference that improved the quality of my life.

I was then thrown a lifeline.

Mom had found an article in the local paper about a CFS rehabilitation program. It was a four-week inpatient rehabilitation program at the Austin Hospital in Melbourne run by Dr. Lionel Lubitz and specifically designed for people with chronic fatigue syndrome. It consisted of a little bit of everything: movement, physical recovery, lifestyle and recreation, counseling, nutrition, and a little bit of cognitive work. It was well structured, and it made sense to me as someone with chronic fatigue syndrome.

It wasn't about pushing the body hard or doing stuff that wasn't helpful. It was ultimately a rehabilitation program for the brain and the body.

My parents and I decided it was worth a shot. Anything was worth a shot.

The program wasn't a "get cured in four weeks" kinda program—it was rehabilitating to have some quality of life. I started the program only being able to do half a pushup on my knees and walking for two minutes. By the end of week four, I could do seventeen pushups and walk for ten minutes.

The team of professionals also helped me work on my brain function and concentration. Over the four weeks, my cognitive function improved, and it also gave me structure to my day. They were strict with sleep/wake/rest times and had regimented mealtimes to give us the best structure and routine for recovery. After three years of doing nothing, I had lost all confidence in myself, but the Austin program showed me that it was possible to live again.

Even though I wasn't completely back to my old self within the four weeks, I realized that I could improve. I had a sense of hope and renewal.

After seeing my strength improve quite dramatically, I remember seeing myself in the mirror after the program and seeing a slight increase in muscle tone and strength that I hadn't seen in years as I was so deconditioned, I lost all my muscle mass over those first three years. I started to believe that one day I would be completely healthy again.

I was keen to maintain my progress, so the team organized a training group for chronic fatigue sufferers who had completed the program. It ran twice a week and was run by Erin Splatt. In a non-threatening, encouraging environment, she reinforced the importance of reconditioning the body and nutrition. She taught us how the body adapts according to the amount of movement we do through progressive overload, and we also worked on our mindset and attitude, which was a gamechanger. It was practical and proactive and not condescending. She didn't say things like: "Think more positively and you will get better."

Instead, it was about how we can be more proactive and how our attitude can shape how we feel. It was all about consistency and accountability, which was the cornerstone of recovery. With a gradual build-up of strength reconditioning and recovery, I started to regain my energy. I was able to cope with more at school, and I was able to hang out with friends again. I attended my Year 12 ball and more importantly, I passed my high school examinations (just).

Of course there were days, and sometimes weeks, where I didn't feel great. But I was determined to help myself get healthy again. It was the small steps I took toward better health that helped me the most. I used to get my dad to take me to the pool before school to do some movement in the water and over time eventually laps—some days I would only last five minutes in the water. But again, I said to myself, *At least I am doing something. I will get stronger eventually if I stick at it.*

Consistency was key!

THE NOT-SO SOCIAL BUTTERFLY

Socializing was another difficult obstacle to overcome—it was such a mind game for me to go out and see my friends. I used to think to myself, *what will happen if I stay out for too long, or if I don't sleep tonight, or if I'm not in bed by 9 p.m.? Will I be sick in bed for two weeks?*

Then there was a secondary social anxiety that I experienced. Fear of judgment from others. *What are they going to think of me?*

What are they going to say? There were lots of doubtful and anxious thoughts going through my mind. On one hand, I was excited to see my friends, and on the other, I was terrified of the consequences if I felt worse.

With support from my family and good friends, I was able to push through that mental barrier and socialize, even if it was only thirty minutes at a time to start with. My confidence grew as I started believing and seeing that I was slowly getting better. It made it easier to try new things again and be proactive about my recovery. Instead of letting chronic fatigue syndrome control me, I started to regain control over my life. Of course, I was lacking in energy, but my strength and stamina started to return and that meant I could do more without feeling worse.

However, even though I had signs of progress with this program, I still believed that *someone* or *something* had to fix me.

A PIECE OF THE ACCEPTANCE PUZZLE

I continued to battle symptoms and wasn't completely sold on the idea that I could get better without a pill or a special doctor. So when we finally got in to see a renowned alternative integrative doctor, we hoped this was the cure. That *he* was the cure. That there was a cure.

This doctor was in demand, and you could only get in to see him if you already knew one of his patients, then there was a four-month wait list and sometimes a two-hour wait in his clinic for your actual appointment. (Not fun when you're suffering from chronic fatigue syndrome.)

I was filled with fear and excitement as I sat in his waiting room. It was our last hope. We'd basically tried everything else, and we were desperate. I was desperate. But our hope was sparked because this doctor had a reputation for fixing the so-called unfixable.

He was small with frizzy white hair that reminded me of Albert Einstein. He wore a white lab coat, which furthered his Nutty Professor look. He was a good man, and he had a deeper mind than anyone else I'd met. There was intensity in his eyes when he looked at me and you could tell he wasn't mucking around.

I did some weird things in the sessions with that doc. He rubbed potions on my skin that he had concocted, and he made me drink the most disgusting mineral liquid that smelled like dog wee. I even drank tea that was from some special bark off a tree. (I was willing to do anything).

The first time I walked into his clinic, within a second of meeting him, he said, "Do you drink Coca Cola, my boy?"

I shyly replied, "Yes, sometimes."

"Get rid of it. It's poison, my boy."

So I did. I was willing to try anything to get better. I laid down on his practice table. He asked me to hum "Happy Birthday" while he tapped up and down my spine for many minutes on end. I thought to myself, *If I have to hum "Happy Birthday" while a doctor taps my back to get my life back…I'll freaking do it!*

Months went on, I had twenty sessions with this doc, and it wasn't cheap. My parents had to chip in (I don't know how they did it, as they weren't wealthy). I'd noticed slight improvements here and there, but nothing really tangible, and it was hard to know what was working and what wasn't. I certainly wasn't feeling significantly better like I expected to be after twenty, two-hour sessions with the nutty professor.

And then came the day.

It was 2:30 p.m. on a Thursday afternoon. My last session with the doctor.

Doc was poking and prodding me and making his special potions. He did all these random alternative tests on my heart and body. In his eyes, these tests determined if I still had chronic fatigue or not. While he did them, he was muttering numbers under his breath. After about a minute of finishing his weird and whacky tests, the moment had finally come; this was my destiny. He looked into my eyes and said, "All right my boy; you don't have chronic fatigue syndrome anymore."

I was struck by two emotions: utter joy and apprehension. On the one hand, I couldn't believe what he was saying, like it felt almost too good to be true. On the other hand, I didn't actually feel much better. Maybe a slight improvement over the twenty sessions, but no crazy amazing change which I was expecting to feel.

I said, "So what do I do now? Can I run?"

At this point, I hadn't been able to run for almost four years. It was the one thing I so badly wanted to do again.

He replied, "Yes, my boy—you can go for a run now."

I was so eager that I walked straight out of his office, across the road to a beautiful oval park. I had longingly watched so many people run across the grass each time I went to the doc's clinic.

I laced up my shoes, took my jumper off and started running. I remember thinking to myself, *this is weird, am I better? I don't feel much different, but if doc said I'm better, I must be better.*

Five minutes into the run, I hit a wall. I went from feeling okay, to not great, to absolutely terrible. I had to lie down on the ground just to muster up the energy to get back to my car and drive home. I got home and crashed into bed.

I was bedridden for another couple of weeks. My symptoms flared and my emotional wellbeing spiraled. I was crippled again with doubt, anger, and sadness.

I was neck-deep in a one-step forward, two-steps back situation. Initially I was upset. *It didn't work*, I said to myself. *I have failed again.* But something special happened during this dark time.

After two weeks of more struggle, the anger and sadness faded…and the day had arrived. An epiphany sparked. A breakthrough.

No one can get you better but you, Toby.

No one can fix you but you.

There is no pill or person that can cure you, but you.

The realization was clear. Bold. Unapologetic. True.

I had spent years searching for someone or something to fix me and it never worked. I invested so much power in everything outside of myself, that I really didn't do much in-between to help myself.

We are brought to believe that if we get sick, we go to the doctor, get blood tests, then take a pill—and the problem will go away.

But in my case, after a truckload of blood tests and pills, antibiotics and trialing different techniques and procedures, I realized that none were the answer.

The answer was me.

While I was spending one to three hours a week on specialists and quick fixes outside of myself, there were still 165 hours per week that I could control. I began to wonder how I could use that time effectively to help myself.

I thought back to when I had made the most progress—the four-week rehabilitation program that was centered around me doing the right things at the right time. It was the small things that made the biggest differences.

Before this realization, I was a major victim of my circumstances. I was really good at throwing a pity party for myself and repeating, "This is so unfair."

But after three years of indescribable suffering and heartache, I was ready for change. I let go of the victim mentality and decided to become a victor.

I didn't know how long the journey would take, but I knew that searching outside of myself to get better wasn't working. It cost a ton of money, it took *a lot* of time and energy and ultimately, it took my hope and nearly my sanity.

The realization that nobody could fix me, but me, gave me real hope for the first time. I felt in control. I was taking full responsibility for my health and life, I felt free.

The cool thing with this newfound responsibility was that I could still be supported by people outside of me, but this time, I wasn't looking to be cured. I was looking for external support from people who knew better than me in their field. But I was the one taking charge of getting better. I took recovery in my hands, fully committed to myself and the process. Mind, body and spirit. From a place of calm, not despair. From a place of hope, not hate. For the first time, it felt really good to be in the driver's seat of my recovery. I would write notes to myself like: *I can get better, I will get better, I am getting better,* and I would read it out loud every day.

I started working on everything recovery related one step at a time. Improving my sleep, dialing in my nutrition, getting the perfect sweet spot with my body's energy output, getting my routine and structure right between activity, rest and expansion. As all this started to take place, my mindset improved dramatically, I started reading personal development books and found mentors and blogs (shout-out to Craig Harper) that inspired me and helped me stay consistent and focused. And ultimately, over time, all of this had a compound effect on my health and well-being. My sleep improved, my gut health got better, my immune system strengthened, my muscle condition started coming up, my stamina and capacity increased, and I was able to do more without feeling worse.

Fast forward a year and I was living again. Living life, socializing, working and having fun. I had a new lease on life.

MY WHY BECOMES REAL

Two years into being sick, during one of my darkest hours, I wrote this down on a piece of paper:

I don't know why this is happening to me, this is so unfair, but I know one day when I get better, I will make sure no one else has to suffer like I did.

This was my why. And now that I felt better, I was going to keep that promise. Thinking about the millions of people in the world suffering, gave me an extraordinary purpose to make sure they didn't have to suffer the way I did. And to show people a way out.

At age nineteen, I invested the only $400 I had into getting a website made up with a blog. This was 2007 when blogs were a thing. I called the website www.cfshealth.com because for me CFS didn't stand for chronic fatigue syndrome anymore, it stood for **Choice, Freedom, Success.** Because that's what I created, and I knew if I could do it, others could do it also.

I enrolled in a health and fitness diploma in Australia as reconditioning my body was paramount to recovery. I learned a lot and was so inspired that I started writing my own program in 2008. Soon after I became qualified, I landed myself a job as a health and fitness coach and within months of starting, I became pretty successful. The difference was I actually cared about people and within twelve months, I was fully booked out and making appointments morning and night.

I loved it. I trained the general population. From kids to teens, adults and the elderly. Because of my own personal journey and my education background, I was able to relate to others and prescribe the appropriate program based on their situation and circumstances.

One thing that going through chronic fatigue syndrome does is it deepens you; it makes you more grounded and empathic. Once you go through something like this, there is no room for small talk. You can relate to almost anyone because of the pain and the suffering. This set me in good stead to train and help pretty much anyone who came to see me.

While I was doing this, I was calling doctors' clinics and knocking on medical clinics doors to connect with and tell doctors that there is a solution for chronic fatigue syndrome recovery and that I was creating a program for it. Most laughed. Who could blame them? I was nineteen and dressed in my dad's suit (that didn't fit me).

About two years later, I grew my health coaching practice and worked with kids on sport-specific training as well as mentoring clients to be the best version of themselves physically and emotionally.

MONEY OR MEANING

At the time, a lot of my clients were very successful people, smart, wise and made a lot of money. Coming from a family who weren't wealthy; I didn't want to have to experience the same.

One day, I woke up and thought, *how am I ever going to be truly successful like my clients as a health coach?* So, I decided I'd become a real estate agent. I loved houses. In fact, even though we didn't have the money to buy them, Mom and I would drive around the local suburb most Saturdays and look at homes together for fun. Plus, I was good at talking to people so I thought real estate would be fun. My boss, who I rented a gym space from, thought I was crazy, but he said if I don't like it, I can come back.

So I went to get my real estate license in my early twenties. It took two weeks and then it was official. I was a licensed real estate agent, and I landed a sales job as an agent the next day: $60,000 plus commission. This was huge almost two decades ago, especially for someone in their twenties. I was over the moon. My dad's suit came in handy again!

But four days later, things took a turn. I was sitting in a boardroom meeting with the directors and all the other agents. It was a quarterly sales meeting, and it was all about the money. Something felt off. I had this gut feeling this wasn't for me. Halfway through the meeting, I had this urge of truth that struck me to my core. I stood up and sheepishly raised my hand as I called out to the head director.

"Damien?"

"Yes, Toby, what's up?" he asked.

"Well I don't think this is for me. This job."

And then, to the shock of Damien and the rest of the sales team, I pushed the chair back, thanked Damien for the four days, and left.

I felt sick to my stomach. Nervous like I was going to throw up. But I had to trust myself and stand in my truth. It all felt like a blur in that office, but walking out, I felt empowered. I knew exactly what my true calling was. I knew I was put on this earth to do something impactful and helping people with chronic fatigue syndrome was more important to me than selling houses. I couldn't ignore it any longer.

ALL-IN ON CFS HEALTH

The very next day, I registered the company CFS Health Centre. I went back to my old health and fitness gym and set up my first proper office. The CFS Health Centre was official, and I knew I'd never give up on this mission to make sure other people didn't have to suffer like I did. As I started up CFS Health Centre, I eventually got in contact with Dr. Lionel Lubitz's office, who was the doctor who helped me with my recovery in that four-week program. I explained to the receptionist that I wanted to book an appointment with Dr. Lubitz to show him my recovery program that I created. He accepted the appointment, and I was so excited to share with him what I came up with because I knew he understood that recovery was possible.

The day of the interview, I was nervous and excited. I thought I better bring him a gift to show my appreciation for him accepting my appointment. I went to the local grocery shop and made a beeline to the confectionery section to get him something nice. There were so many choices, and it was hard to know what chocolate to buy for a doctor. Then out of the corner of my eye

I saw part of my name on that yellow Toblerone bar. I thought, *ah that's an omen.*

I drove an hour to get to Dr. Lionel Lubitz's offices in the Royal Children's Hospital. It was a special day for me, as five years prior, I was there for being sick and now I was walking in as a healthy person about to share my big vision for the future to make the world a better place. With the Toblerone bar in one hand and my program outlay in the other, I was ready.

"Toby Morrison, you may come in now, Dr. Lubitz is ready to see you," said the receptionist.

When I walked into his office, Dr. Lubitz said, "Toby, my god look at you, big and strong, you look great! Please sit down and tell me what I can do for you today."

"Firstly Lionel, I want to thank you for letting me share this with you, here is a little gift."

As I handed over the Toblerone, he said, "How did you know this is the only chocolate I actually eat?"

I knew right then and there this meeting was going to be a success. We sat down and I told him my big vision and shared all the program details and how it would work. He loved it.

But with one minor tweak—make the program longer.

While I had designed the program for over four weeks, he explained that an out-patient program needed to be longer in order for patients to make true tangible progress. He was right of course, so I extended the program out longer to account for the fact that recovery takes time. I drove home that day with a smile as wide as my ears.

REAL-LIFE HELP WITH REAL-LIFE PEOPLE

I continued with my current clients but it was time to finally help people with chronic fatigue syndrome. The next week, I got a call from my neighbor.

"Hey Toby, my friend Ash has CFS, and he doesn't know what to do. I explained how you got better. Would you be able to help him?"

The answer was of course, yes.

I called Ash later that day and explained that I might not have all the answers, but I knew I could help him rebuild his health. We scheduled a time and had our first session. It was hard. He was in a very bad way. He couldn't believe that he had to deal with chronic fatigue syndrome. He was so enraged and upset about his current situation, as he had gone from being an elite sportsman to not being able to run at all. During our first session, he mainly expressed how pissed off he was about the fact he couldn't run.

In that session, we set some foundations, but there was no point really putting much into practice because I knew that until he accepted his current situation, he wouldn't be able to move forward. So that day, I lent an ear. I listened and sympathized with him, as I truly understood what he was going through.

To my surprise, the next seven sessions were focused on mindset because not accepting his current reality was actually halting his recovery. He was constantly beating himself up and in total victim mode. It wasn't until session eight that he had a breakthrough and finally reached acceptance. I reassured him that acceptance isn't resignation and in fact it's the starting point of his recovery because now he can focus all his energy and attention on where he is at right now.

From that week on, Ash showed up differently. He showed up more relaxed and with a can-do attitude. He was no longer his worst enemy. In just twelve weeks, he started to notice positive changes. Less brain fog. Less pain. Better sleep. Better baseline. Less energy dips. Feeling better about life in general. He was able to move more, start structured movement sessions, and wake up most days feeling better than he did the previous twelve months. He started to notice glimpses of energy coming back.

Six months later, after diligently working with me, he was back running as part of his progression plan. We slowly integrated short runs into his weekly structure and routine. The day he was able to start jogging again, he wore a big smile the whole time.

I felt so proud and excited for him. When he left my office, I thought, *this really works*! And it didn't just work for me, but for others too. Watching it play out in front of my very own eyes was validating and exciting.

Twelve months later, he was able to go back to running at a professional level.

A few days after Ash started, another person reached out for help in regards to CFS. Her mother called me and explained that she was the director of health and medicine across seven hospitals in Australia. Her daughter, Bec, had CFS and they'd heard that I'd made a recovery and wanted to speak with me.

Claire said, "We have tried everything Toby. *Everything*. You are our last hope."

I explained to her that recovery isn't a quick fix cure but a process. And that I don't get anyone better, I guide people to help themselves get healthy and start living again.

When Bec came to see me at the health center, she was overwhelmed. Both her and Claire had no idea what to do, but they were open to anything. So, I set her up first and foremost with a suitable baseline so she wasn't under or overdoing it. *(We talk about baselines later so stay tuned)*. We looked at her sleep/wake cycles, her daily nutrition and rest/activity ratios.

After four weeks of figuring out and adjusting a few things, relief started to happen in more ways than one. Firstly, Bec seemed calmer and held almost a graceful attitude towards recovery versus a resistance to it. Secondly, her body started to respond really well to the baseline we created around her current capacity. Things became more doable.

Thirdly, and what I found interesting, was the change with her mom (and caregiver), Claire. On the fourth week of working together, Claire confided in me. She said, "Toby, thank you so much. Do you know what the biggest help is for me? I can finally just be a mom again. I am no longer the coach or the carer."

She went on to say that she of course would continue to support her, but that it was a relief to have just one role rather than many. It really improved their relationship.

Six months on, Bec was thriving with her recovery. Twelve months later, she was stronger than ever and doing proper gym sessions, studying, and exploring work options.

Here's what was interesting—as Bec got healthy and started to live again, she stayed as a client for many years. Not because she needed me, but because she loved the accountability, the coaching, the support, and most importantly, she knew it was an investment that gave her more than money could buy...*life*.

Today, she is healthy and no longer has CFS. She went on to become a paramedic and now saves lives for a living. Bec is an example of what recovery can be like.

I like to remind people that **health is forever, but recovery doesn't have to be.**

FULL-CIRCLE

After working with Ash and Bec, word of mouth spread and within six months, I had people of all ages seeing me for their CFS. It was such an exciting time for me because I fell in love with the potential that each client had. Although they felt like their life was over, I knew their life was just beginning. I documented every single client's journey. I studied what worked and what didn't work, and I took notes every evening before I finished work and my filing cabinet started to fill.

Clients were noticing positive changes, and I tracked their progress over the weeks. I started writing a book based on the data and information I was collecting directly from the clients, and two years later, I published my first book *Chronic Fatigue Syndrome: A Guide to Recovery*.

Soon I became known across Australia, and others started recommending me to people they knew with CFS. Within months, I was fully booked. Not only that, but within twelve months, I had people driving and flying interstate to come and do my program; one came all the way from London. The following years, I had a client fly me to Dubai and France to help them get better. The day before I flew to France, I headed to my local cafe for one more breakfast in Australia and you wouldn't believe who was at the cafe. It was Damien Kelly, the director of the real estate firm I quit five years prior.

He greeted me with a smile, "Toby, I remember you! What are you up to these days?"

"Well, you wouldn't believe it, Damien, but the next day after I quit real estate, I opened up my own company called CFS Health to do what I'm passionate about which is to help people with chronic fatigue syndrome get healthy again."

"Wow that's cool, how's it going?" he asked.

"It's going great, I am helping lots of people get their life back, I've written a book, and tomorrow I am being flown to France to help a client."

His jaw dropped. He couldn't believe my reality.

"Holy shit, Toby, that's incredible. You are really living the dream." He put his hand out and shook mine with pride.

Talk about a full-circle moment.

Since walking out on that job, I went on to do things I never thought was possible. I have traveled the world, coached over 5,500 people in 78 countries over the last fifteen years, scuba-dived the Great Barrier Reef, snow boarded, and surfed seriously big waves in Fiji called Frigates and Cloudbreak.

These days, I spend my time between being the founder of CFS Health, helping my incredible team and clients achieve their life's goals and dreams. Most days, I am down at the beach surfing or in the gym training, hanging out with my dog Ziggy, traveling the world to see new cultures and see friends, and finding new beautiful nature spots. I love surfing, training, nature, kayaking, yoga, Tai Chi, bathing in the sun, art, and trying new things, like building a shack and even playing piano.

I know that life with CFS makes you feel helpless, restless, frustrated, sad, angry, weak, miserable, and uncertain about the future. But I also know there's a life beyond CFS that is waiting for you. One full of possibilities.

I have seen recovery success happen way too many times for so many people, that I know it's possible for you too. From the most severe types with a long list of other chronic health conditions to the milder symptoms and more semi-functioning. People regain their health and quality of life, and they go on to fully living again.

This book will show you the exact CFS Health frameworks these people used to recover. But before we do, we must cover some important fundamentals. As my builder friend Tom says, "If you want a quality home, you must first build a strong foundation to create the quality home you want." The same goes for your health and recovery.

TAKEAWAYS

You are the answer to your own recovery. You
are the miracle you're searching for.

No matter what remedies, fixes, or specialists
you have tried before, the journey isn't
over. There is hope on the horizon.

The journey of trying everything and anything is
common, but it's not necessary once you know
the strategies and start to build a foundation.

Doing the right thing at the right time
is vital to your recovery.

RECOVERY INSPIRATION

Watch my full personal story here on how
I healed from CFS after 4.5 hard years.

CHAPTER 3

Getting Into the Green Zone

When I was going through CFS, there were four specific phases I went through in order to get to the other side of recovery. At the time I had no idea there were phases, but now, after working with thousands of people, I have realized every single person who gets better from CFS has to go through these four specific phases to get to the other side of recovery.

I call it the **Four Levels of Recovery Readiness.**

But before we deep dive into those four levels, I want to share with you some personal insights I've observed over the decades. I'm not saying these are scientific facts; I am just sharing the interesting themes I have noticed, and I can assure you my research has been extensive.

Observation 1—It's not laziness

I have observed that CFS isn't an illness that affects lazy people. I have never met a person who had chronic fatigue syndrome who was lazy. Period. It affects doers, people who do great things, people who want to conquer the world, people who try to get the most out of themselves and life. Not people who want to sit around and do nothing with their lives. Around 80% of people I work with on a daily basis are type A personalities. They have high standards or are perfectionists of some sort.

Observation 2—It's not one thing

Almost everyone I have met with chronic fatigue syndrome attributes a combination of factors to getting sick in the first place. These factors typically include: viruses, infections, overtraining, prolonged mental or emotional stress, trauma, pushing their bodies for too long, and environmental stresses like exposure to chemicals or mold.

For me personally, it was glandular fever ("mono"), overtraining (not listening to my body and recovering appropriately from glandular fever) and prolonged emotional and mental stress that was the perfect recipe for CFS to transpire. This is a great recipe for the brain and body to eventually go into shut down mode. For some, it's a gradual decline to ill health and for others the onset can be fast.

Observation 3—It's no one's fault

Most people with chronic fatigue syndrome are hyper-responsible about their situation. They don't want to be sick; it's the last thing in the world that they want. When your life feels like it has been taken from you, it is easy to fall into the guilt and shame cycle. Please give yourself some grace here, the situation you are in is not your fault. Most people I meet from around the world have been left in what I call the medical desert. They are searching for answers from a medical system that doesn't have any. They are victims of a system that does not have a metric or a tried-and-tested way to handle CFS. They are caught in between the cracks of a system that does not have a firm or holistic grounding for treating CFS.

Observation 4—It's counterintuitive to conditioning

It's common for people with CFS to search and search outside themselves for answers. They are not lazy people but very proactive about finding solutions. It's normal for us to believe and expect a solution, after all as children, we are brought up to believe that if you get sick, you go to the doctor, perhaps get something from the doctor, and then you get better. Unfortunately, that doesn't work for chronic fatigue syndrome. And that's a huge curveball. It's counterintuitive to the conditioning most of us were raised in. While some of these external supplementary aids may be useful and sometimes helpful, they are certainly not the answer to a bigger problem. But we have been taught that the medical system will have the answers—so when they don't, we feel lost and alone. CFS sufferers are only wanting to be well and live well. They will search anywhere for relief. Finding the path to recovery means going against the conditioning we were raised in.

**People with chronic illnesses aren't faking being sick.
They are actually faking being well.**

THE FOUR LEVELS
OF RECOVERY READINESS

When it comes to chronic fatigue syndrome and recovery, there are four levels you must pass through to come out the other end and ultimately regain your health and life again. It's important to recognize which level you are currently in. It's also important to say that none of these zones/levels are wrong or right. They just are. You might relate to being in all four. Or maybe you have been stuck on a specific one. There is no judgment with this, no matter where you are, awareness is the first step to change. In order to get better you have to move up to level four eventually.

Red: The Giving Up Zone

We've all been there. This is where you believe recovery is simply not possible for you. You know that there are people around the world that have gotten better, but you believe you never will. You think you've tried everything, and that nothing works. You believe that there are no options left. In this zone you complain a lot and you blame others regularly because you feel stuck. You often think, *What's the point?* when you are in the red zone. It's also common and appropriate to feel a sense of fear and isolation here.

In the red zone you may say things like:

"What's the point?"

"Will this ever end?"

"This is too hard. I will never get better."

Amber: The Hoping Zone

You begin to believe it's possible to get better; you just don't know how. You still feel lost and overwhelmed. In the hoping zone, you regularly pray or wish for a miracle to happen, only to wake up in the morning and realize that nothing has changed. You feel lost, constantly guessing and self-sabotaging (that is, not doing the right things to improve your situation). You feel like you're going around and around in circles. You're hoping for something to change, but you're ultimately still waiting for that to happen.

In the amber zone you may say things like:

"I just need a miracle."

"I'm praying for something to change."

"Nothing has changed."

Light Green: The Seeking Zone

As we move up, this is where things feel a little more exciting, yet that excitement often ends with a sense of despair. You know you can get better, but you believe that you need someone or something to fix you. If you are in the seeking zone, you feel like you are just coping. You're feeling consumed by everything you try, whether that be a new health guru or the next whiz-bang high-tech device that has come out.

Here, you might go down a rabbit hole of Doctor Google, searching for a million different modalities that can make all the symptoms go away. This is where you might have twenty window tabs open on your computer, hoping to find the answer to your problems. In this zone, you're trying quick fix strategies. If you're in the seeking zone, you will be feeling very tested here. You'll have research-seeking fatigue on top of your chronic fatigue syndrome exhaustion. The cognitive overload is real.

There's a point in the seeking zone where you get fed up with it and you start to believe that you might have to settle. You often feel like you're back down to the giving up zone. It's a scary place, but often feels like a safer place, particularly after being let down so many times. It feels safer than being let down yet again by another quick fix remedy.

In the light green zone, you may say things like:

"Maybe I should try…[insert new remedy]"

"Maybe I could see that new doctor."

"This tech device sounds amazing, maybe it will fix it."

"Will the search ever end?"

Green: The Owning Zone

This is where you start to realize that the body does heal itself when you do the right things at the right times. You finally wake up and realize that no one else will fix you, but you.

Instead of feeling sad about that, you feel liberated. You feel free for the first time, and you finally feel true possibility because you are taking your health and your recovery into your own hands. No longer are you hoping or wishing. Instead, you're in the driver's seat of your recovery. In the owning zone, you start to have an inner certainty that you didn't have before. You ultimately start to take ownership and responsibility of your health and life one step at a time. You start to be self-led instead of being led by the health system and the culture of taking a pill and getting better. And here you start to become truer to yourself. At CFS Health, we call this the "true you."

In the green zone you may say things like:

"I'm getting better each day."

"I can do this."

"I let go of the past."

"I'm building my new future."

"I'm being true to myself."

"I don't need to search anymore."

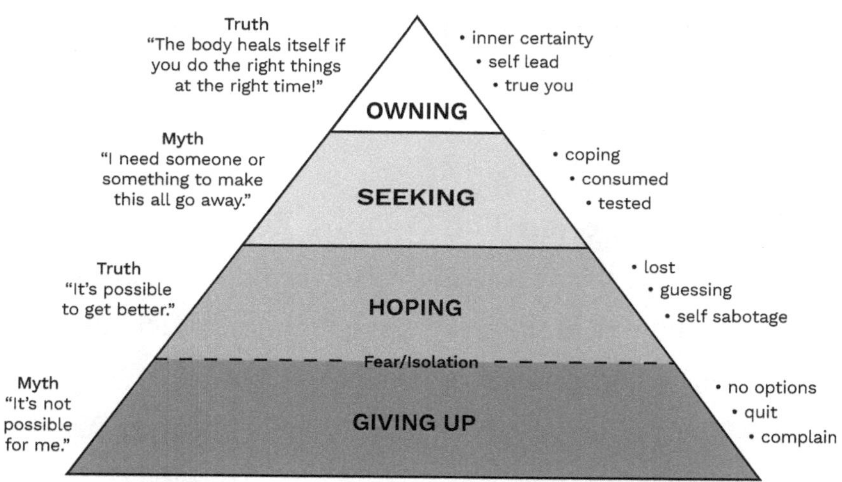

THE ZONE FLUX

Through the years, I've witnessed so many people go through these four zones, and it's pretty damn cool to see people move from giving up to reaching the owning zone stage. The difference is night and day.

Charlie was one such person who experienced the difference; it was night and day (but it didn't happen overnight!).

Charlie wears many hats—former nurse, mother, wife and community-oriented citizen. When she first enrolled in our flagship Recovery Mentorship Program in 2018, she went from bed, to the sofa, and back to bed. Life wasn't good. She was at her wit's end. Although she enjoyed sipping tea, she was sick and tired of doing that in bed watching the world go by. She desperately wanted to get better.

She was also suffering with deep "mother-guilt" for not being able to do all the things she wanted to do with her children. This compounded her symptoms and impacted her mental health. Like most people, she wanted to get better yesterday. The anger, frustration and lack of self-compassion spun like a vicious cycle of anguish that she couldn't exit. She had been suffering for years so who could blame her.

She had tried everything. She'd done the endless doctors' rounds, the 'get better quick' schemes, the healthcare system, and the alternative route. All with not much luck or support. Charlie started to believe she was "a hopeless case."

She contacted CFS Health as a last resort. I remember our first phone call. She was super frustrated. She said things like:

"When is this going to end, Toby?"

"I just don't understand why I have to feel this way."

"It's so unfair."

"Is it even possible for me to get better?"

"I can't even be there for my kids. What sort of mother am I?"

Although my heart sank for Charlie's situation, I was full of optimism. I knew her life was going to change. Sure, she was at a loss. But she was smack in the middle of the Giving Up zone and that's how it feels when you're there. Defeated. Agonizing, Hopeless.

But luckily for Charlie, zones are not stations we stop at, they are places we move through. I highlighted to Charlie that she was in the Giving Up zone.

"Damn, right I am." she said.

We started there. Right where she was. Right where she needed to be fully met. But certainly not where we intended her to stay.

Charlie and I worked together for around two years in our Online Mentorship Program. Early on it was tough, it was as if a dark cloud of heaviness followed her around daily. Her motivation levels were extremely low, her secondary depression and anxiety kicked in, and her frustration was at an all-time high.

She remained deeply rooted in the Giving Up Zone, not because she didn't want any other zone but because she was simply trying to function. But I knew there was hope. That there were other zones on the horizon for her to experience. But for change to happen, change had to happen. Charlie had to be that change. But I promised her that I would coach her through.

There were five things we did to help Charlie turn her recovery around. We needed to accept that she was in the Giving Up Zone and that it was a phase not a permanent state.

1. Mindset of acceptance

I encouraged Charlie to work on her mindset. To accept her situation and know what phase she was in. We had to stop the pity party, as hard as it was. She felt like everything was out of her control (which a lot of it was). But Charlie needed to sit back into the driver's seat and steer her recovery. She needed to deliberately focus on what she could do and what she could control. I challenged Charlie to get the facts straight—that recovery was possible, and that going from victim to victor, from complexity to calm, was the first step in the right direction.

It was a challenge to shift for her but not changing was causing more distress so she decided to go all in and move the needle in her mind: from hopeless to hopeful.

2. Find her baseline

We stopped her push-crash cycle by finding her baseline (which you will learn all about in the next chapter). This enabled her to stabilize her energy levels and moods. She stopped having crazy ups and downs and became calmer. This decreased her stress dramatically.

3. Sleep

We also improved her sleep quality by setting up a proper routine and structure. She had irregular sleep patterns, and it was sabotaging her. She would sometimes sleep through the day and then not be able to sleep at night. Her sleep was erratic and created erratic outcomes.

4. Habits

We implemented new recovery habits that set the foundation for progress to happen. We looked at her nutrition and replaced highly processed and sugary foods with more protein and whole foods. This stopped her blood sugar levels crashing a lot throughout the day.

5. Progress over time

We implemented a progress and maintenance plan so as she progressed we could allow enough time for her body to adapt appropriately to the stimulus we provided. This allowed Charlie to progress in a step-by-step way and increase her energy levels appropriately. Now this didn't happen overnight. We made these changes incrementally according to the way Charlie's body adapted and responded.

Over the coming months Charlie started to make progress. Not a lot at the start, but enough for her to see that it was working. Now, guess what happened? You bet ya! Charlie got out of the Giving Up Zone, she went through the Hoping Zone, upgraded to the Seeking Zone, and eventually went into the Owning Zone.

I watched Charlie go from feeling sad and hopeless, to strong, confident, and self-led. She went from mumbling with her head down and dreading the future, to speaking with confidence and looking forward to her future. Her smile and laughter came back.

Charlie got better and she got her life back! She's an amazing wife, mother and now a mentor with CFS Health. The crazy thing is, even her husband Justin said he feels like he got a new wife. Pretty cool right! They ended up buying an old farm in the UK countryside. She is busy renovating the farmhouse, mentoring others, and spending time with family. What a legend!

Looking from the outside, it's easy to think that Charlie had a miraculous recovery, almost as if luck was on her side. But you can see this wasn't luck, it was strategy. Charlie did the right things at the right times to get the right results over time.

There's only one type of luck I believe in, which I learned from the great holistic health coach, Paul Chek. Which is—luck stands for…**L**abour, **U**nder, **C**orrect, **K**nowledge.

If it's possible for Charlie and thousands of people I have seen get better, it's possible for you too.

Believe it or not, Charlie flew all the way to Australia to do an in-person interview to share all the details on how she got her life back. Listen to Charlie's inspirational recovery story here:

Now, before you worry about how long you may have been in the red, amber or light green zone. Don't be concerned, I'm not writing this book to keep you in those zones—reading this book is the gateway to moving into the Owning Zone.

And yes, that zone is not a pipe dream; it's very possible for you.

Charlie isn't an anomaly. This isn't a book about depicting "exceptions to the rule"; it's a tried-and-tested method for success for anyone.

Take Stephanie for example. Stephanie was sixteen years old when her mom contacted us. Stephanie wasn't interested in doing our program. She was exasperated from working with so-called "experts" and feeling a sense of doom when "nothing worked."

Stephanie was neck-deep in the Giving Up zone and saw us the next expert team "doomed to fail."

Fair enough I thought. She had tried countless things, people and programs. *Who could blame her for feeling that way?* For being pessimistic about the future. Luckily, Stephanie had a warrior mom who refused to join her in the Giving Up zone. She encouraged (and pleaded) for Stephanie to join our program.

Stephanie spent the entire first session disengaged. Her head was down and she didn't participate. She was more interested in looking at the ground than at us. But we didn't mind. We understood that Stephanie was reluctant to feel hope when she had been hopeful about a myriad of other things that never worked out. Stephanie was just trying to protect herself from disappointment and hurt.

The next session started the same. Head down, no engagement or eye contact.

About halfway through the session, one of our CFS team members said…"and doing our program means no more false promises, no more pills or magic potions."

Stephanie looked up for the first time. A hint of possibility entered her eyes.

The coach continued, "…and it also means that we encourage you to move from being a victim of this condition to being victorious in YOUR life…whatever that looks like to you."

Stephanie heard truth not false hope. Why? Because she was surrounded by mentors who once suffered from CFS and now were sharing their stories with her. For the first time she was understood. And not just understood but supported. And not just supported by those in her family without CFS, but those who were not in her family who had come out the other side.

Stephanie had a tribe. A community of support who understood her.

Within twelve weeks Stephanie moved from the Giving Up zone to the Hoping zone and then fast-tracked to the Owning zone. She started to feel like herself again, and she felt like she had a plan to get out of this for the first time in her recovery and it felt good! She painted her nails as a reflection of her mood and she would come and show me her colored nails, flashing around her bright pinks, oranges and reds with joy. She started netball again and was filled with the youthful exuberance of a fun-loving sixteen-year-old.

Fast-forward a decade, Stephanie is now an exercise physiologist and a CFS mentor at CFS Health. She remains full of energy and is busy living her best life.

TAKEAWAYS

CFS commonly affects driven, Type A personalities who push themselves too hard. It's linked to factors like viral infections, overtraining, prolonged stress, and environmental exposures.

THE FOUR LEVELS OF RECOVERY READINESS INVOLVES MOVING THROUGH FOUR ZONES.

RED ZONE: Feeling hopeless and stuck, believing recovery is impossible.

AMBER ZONE: Hoping for recovery but feeling lost and overwhelmed.

LIGHT - GREEN ZONE: Actively seeking external solutions but facing frustration and cognitive overload.

GREEN ZONE: Owning the recovery process by taking control and realizing that healing comes from within.

LONG-TERM PERSPECTIVE: Recovery from CFS is not luck but a strategy and gradual process that requires consistent effort, mindset changes, and adaptation over time, as demonstrated by Charlie's experience in the recovery program.

RECOVERY INSPIRATION

Watch Stephanie's full recovery interview here.
Be prepared to be very inspired!

CHAPTER 4

The 3 Stages of Recovery

Two years into my recovery, my family and I went on a recovery spending spree (or maybe that's a searching spree). We tried absolutely *everything*. One of the 100 things we tried that year (not joking) was physiotherapy/personal training. The doctor said I needed to try exercising, so we searched for a professional.

The trainer we went to was smart, very dedicated, and an extremely fit and healthy man. I did a one-on-one session in his personal training studio. I was feeling really weak, nervous, and apprehensive about the whole thing, but I was willing to give anything a go at this stage. We explained to him that I hadn't been well for a while now, and that I was extremely deconditioned with very little strength or energy.

He smiled and said, "No worries, I got you covered."

I will never forget our first session. He walked around in his short shorts and tight shirt with huge quad muscles and biceps popping out like Popeye. I was already feeling weak and nervous, so imagine my reaction when he started the session with a big Swiss ball. He got me to lay over the top of it and walk my hands out on the floor into a pushup position, all while keeping my feet on the ball, not falling off...and then do a pushup. I could barely do the walk out bit, let alone the pushups. My whole body was shaking. I could almost see myself rolling off the ball and face-planting into the floor.

I somehow got through the first twenty minutes of that session, but I didn't feel great. At the end, he did some deep tissue work on my legs, massaging them and pressing into trigger points. I'm not sure what was more painful, the pushups on the Swiss ball or his elbows digging deep into my deconditioned hamstrings. It felt like a jackhammer thrusting into my muscles and hitting the bone. Mr *"No worries, I've got you covered"* was certainly doing his thing.

Strangely, I assumed it was good for me because he was a professional and the specialist doctor said it would be good for me.

For the next five days I could barely walk! My legs were throbbing from the intense elbow grinds and exercise. I remained sore FOR DAYS! And not good sore either. (I'll cover good soreness vs the bad soreness in the chapter 9.)

That session made me feel shit. Back then, I had no idea that there are 3 stages of recovery, and the level of output someone should do for recovery is dependent on which stage you are in. Turns out I was doing stage 3 activities with stage 3 energy outputs when my body was still in stage 1 of healing and stage 1 energy levels.

As the founder of Apple Steve Jobs once said, "You can only connect the dots by looking backwards." *Yep, I hear ya Steve.*

THE 3 STAGES OF RECOVERY

After connecting the dots and realizing that recovery was a continuum and there was a way to avoid the crash-and-burn moments, and after seeing the evidence of watching thousands of people get healthy and start living again, I developed the 3 Stages of Recovery model.

The model outlines where you're at in *your* recovery and what you need to do based on *your* level. It's a game-changer!

The 3 stages are:

1. The Restore Stage
2. The Re-strengthen Stage
3. The Re-integration Stage

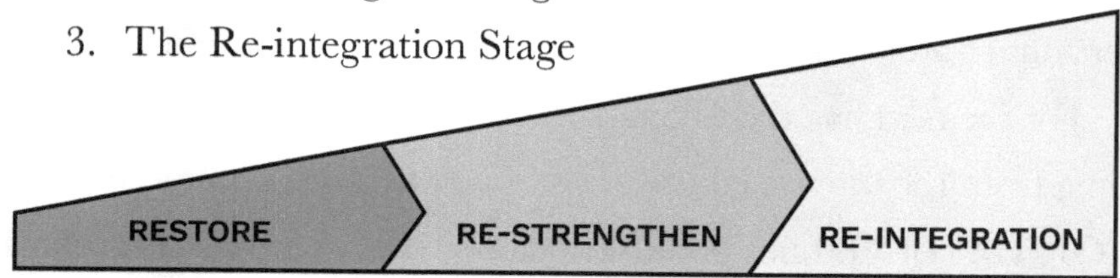

They each have signature characteristics that you can identify and they act as building blocks according to your needs.

Stage 1: Restore (Acute suffering phase)

This is where your body and mind are exhausted almost all the time.

Symptoms are extreme and it feels like you're suffering 24/7. *Note to self:* This is not the stage to visit a PT and do a 1:1 intense exercise session with trigger-point massage.

The most important thing to do in stage 1 is to **restore energy and equilibrium in the body.** Why? Because it's necessary to stabilize your health. Without stability you suffer. Without stability, there is no foundation. Without a foundation you cannot progress. Just like building a great house. Houses that fall apart have unstable foundations. Houses that last forever are built on solid foundations. The same is true for recovery.

The biggest mistake most people make when they're in stage 1 is pushing way beyond their means and trying to force progress too fast. They end up pushing too hard and crashing even harder, often going one step forward and three steps back. It can feel like a never-ending cycle of push-and-crash, push-and-crash! It ends badly and you feel defeated.

In this stage, you should *not* do any form of macro (big) structured exercise or movement. You are usually sleeping anywhere from 12 to 18 hours per day, or at least you are in bed for that amount of time and you are barely functioning.

In stage 1, you don't want to put any strain or added pressure on your brain or body: physically, cognitively or emotionally. It's not that exercise or movement is bad, but it is often prescribed at the wrong time or at the wrong level of intensity and this can actively hinder recovery. Does this sound familiar to you?

In stage 1, you want to have a *less-is-more* approach so you can restore energy and build reserves to create stability and a foundation to build on.

The less is more approach is not about doing nothing and waiting to get better. (Because you can't rest or wait yourself to recovery). Instead you have to start where you are at now in your recovery so you can get better later. In the coming chapters you'll understand exactly what that looks like in the key areas of recovery.

Remember stage 1 is about building a healthy foundation.

Stage 2: Restrengthen (Reconditioning phase)

This is where the body switches out of the acute phase of suffering and instead starts restoring energy in the body. Once there is stability in your recovery (meaning you stop pushing and crashing all the time) you can slowly start to transition into the re-strengthen stage. This stage is all about building strength, stamina, and capacity—physically and cognitively—for where you are at right now in your recovery. This is how progress will begin, albeit in small doses.

The restrengthen stage is where we can start to restrengthen the body appropriately based on where it's at, as your brain and body start to come back online and are figuring out how to use energy again.

Our job here is to figure out the correct amount of energy output and input needed to stop pushing and crashing and also build capacity in the body over time. Once you stabilize, you are literally reconditioning your body and brain back to good health. Think of it as building your capacity gradually over time. This is where it becomes possible to do more appropriate structured energy activities, including both physical and cognitive abilities.

As your capacity grows, your energy output becomes bigger. Meaning you can do more without feeling worse than you currently do. That's kinda great news, right? Doing more without feeling worse. That is what building capacity is all about. But wait…there's more…

Stage 3: Re-integration
(Lifestyle integration phase)

This is where the fun begins. When you start to re-integrate back into life on all levels, including physically, cognitively, emotionally and even spiritually. This is the sexy stage that everyone dreams of, but you can't get there without going through stage 1 and 2 first.

Pro tip: Most people try to skip stage 1 and 2 and live in stage 3 *before* they're ready. They wonder why they're not getting better and they keep going around in circles. If that is you then it's time to take your recovery seriously and fully commit to the process so you can enjoy stage 3 without regressing. Lasting change is not a fleeting moment of feeling like you have your old life back and then having it crumble the next day because you over did it and feel horrible.

Ultimately here, **you're aiming to increase capacity in all areas of that life that matter to you**. Amazing, right?

Not necessarily all at once, but over time. It's about appropriately easing back into and building a life that you love.

The good news is you integrate the lessons from all three stages, and over time you unlock the ultimate guidepost for your health and life, which we call *body wisdom.*

Body wisdom means knowing what to do and when the right time to do it is.

You become familiar with how your body is feeling and what it needs, in other words, knowing when to slow down, when to push forwards, and when to maintain the same level. It's what helps you avoid injury, burnout, recover from colds and flus faster.

You will bounce between all three throughout your recovery. Stages are transitional, meaning they are not black and white. You can slowly transition out of stage 1 into stage 2, and stage 2 to stage 3. There will be times when you feel like you need to rest, there will be times where you feel you can have a lower energy output and times where you feel you can do more in terms of output.

<hr>

**The most important thing is not where
you're at but being able to understand
what you need and when.**

<hr>

As you start to progress, you will expand your capacity, meaning your brain and body get better at adapting to energy output (stimulus big and small)—and you also get better at restoring energy faster.

The purpose of the three stages framework is to simply manage, progress and expand your health and life appropriately based on where you are currently at.

It is the framework that can guide your wellbeing so that you don't get stuck in the push-crash lifecycle where you can't gauge what your body and mind need. It's okay to rest when you need it, but it's equally important to recognize when you have the capacity to exert appropriate energy for where you are at, and in doing so improve your health and keep building your capacity.

Now, often energy is the last thing to come back during recovery. That means that we're *not* using energy as a "progress marker" in recovery initially. The focus needs to be on being able to do more without feeling any worse than you currently do. Meaning you build your capacity (strength and stamina) and as you do that, energy starts to return.

ANNABEL

Many years ago, I had a client named Annabel. At her first appointment with me, I took her through a self-health evaluation. It turned out her biggest problem was knowing how much to do. She had been struggling for years and was neck-deep in stage 1. But Annabel was living as if she were in stage 2 and

3 of recovery and wondering why she wasn't getting anywhere. She was trying to do 30-minute gym sessions, play tennis, and run, and she found herself smashed afterwards. She was going waaaay beyond her capacity and wasn't ready for that yet.

In our first session, I pulled the level of exercise right back. In fact, I told her we were replacing the word "exercise" with the word "movement." *Restorative movement* to be exact.

I asked her to do an easy 5-minute movement routine; a series of guided movements to restore energy. She looked at me weirdly but went into the movements. As she was doing the easy movements I prescribed her, I would stop her *before* she got to the point where her body was struggling and ask her to stop and chill.

I gauged these points by using cues in the stability of her muscles (ensuring she was not getting to the point of shaking or struggling), the tempo of her breathing (keeping it relatively relaxed), and the neutrality of her facial expressions (monitoring for signs of strain or discomfort). You can usually tell if someone is pushing too hard if their face goes all red, sweaty or they start making funny faces as they perform the movement. There's nothing wrong with that as you get healthier; however, in stage 1, we want to avoid that exertion and focus on restorative actions.

After the new shortened routine finished, I said, "Okay Annabel, that's enough."

She looked at me shocked. "What, that's it?"

"Yep, that's perfect for today."

"But I am not even tired or in pain yet. I can do more."

I laughed and said, "That's the point. The reason you haven't been able to make any progress is because you're pushing too hard and then crashing out, and we need to help your body adapt appropriately to the stimulus we give it. And right now, we are giving your body the appropriate amount of stimulus that it can handle. Each week, we will build it up appropriately until your capacity strengthens."

The penny dropped.

"Ahhhh I see," she remarked. "So I don't need to push myself to the point of pain to get the most out of it?"

"That's right. You need to nurture your body by restoring energy, not depleting it to the point where you have nothing left in the tank. You need to stop *before* you feel worse and definitely stop before you're in pain."

She said, "I thought the only way to exercise or to get the most out of a workout was to do it 100%…to push myself."

I smiled and reassured her, "No, that's why you are here with me now; so we can stop that!"

She beamed. Something finally made sense to her.

Like all my clients, I made sure Annabel had a holistic focus, we focused on factors like nutrition and sleep and integrated things carefully along the journey. But the long story short is that in the first 6 months, she went from 5 minutes of restorative movement a day to building her capacity to 25 minutes a day, on top of increasing her cognitive abilities and emotional ones too. Things like reading, writing, and socializing all increased over time.

Within a year, she was back playing tennis and running and this all came from a series of consistent improvements that led to her quality of life being restored. It's been several years since Annabel did the program, but now she's traveling the world, working full time, and living her best life.

HOLISTIC HEALTH HEALS

Once you get the recovery process in place and implement routines that are conducive to healing, the rest takes care of itself. That is of course provided you remain consistent over time, not overnight. My philosophy is—progress over perfection and consistency over intensity gets the results.

**Starting where you are
is critical to success.**

Even if a healthy young person walked into a gym for the first time, no personal trainer would put them on the same plan as someone who had been going to the gym for a year, or even six weeks. If they did, they would likely injure themselves, have delayed onset muscle soreness for days after, and feel depleted after the session. Every single person has to start small and build that muscle, strength and stamina over time, but the difference comes with the starting point. You must start where you're at.

The reason this sometimes feels unnatural for people with CFS is because it's hard to come to terms with the fact that the capacity they have now is so far below what they used to be able to do. Remember my story? I was hooked on being like my old self that I couldn't let go of the person I used to be. And this hindered my progress. I wanted to be the fit unstoppable basketball player that I used to be but reality was I was the deconditioned young man who got puffed tying his shoe laces.

But this is where acceptance comes into play—once you've reached acceptance about the fact your capacity is low, you can start building it up. If you're in a state of denial and continue to do the exercise or activities that you did before you got CFS, that are not appropriate for you right now, you will continually crash and burn.

Recovery can feel like such a long game that you feel it's too much. But recovery is not forever, it just has to be your focus now. Your diagnosis doesn't have to be a life sentence.

Once you get healthy and start to live again, you're not focusing on recovery, you're focusing on life! It's a complete shift.

HOLISTIC HEALTH IS NEVER "ONE THING"

CFS doesn't discriminate—it takes down the best of us. It affects every aspect of life; therefore a multi-faceted approach is needed. I have never met one person who has recovered from CFS (and I have met thousands) who said it was just "one thing" that helped them get better. It's *never* just "one thing."

Most people come to CFS Health once they've tried almost everything. From pills, potions, supplements, specialists, and even weird and whacky therapies.

Now don't get me wrong, many holistic modalities and treatments can be useful, but supplements won't cure your CFS. Medications can be useful for some people, whereas others get more out of brain retraining or breathwork. But it's rarely "one thing" that helps people heal.

This is why we have a comprehensive approach that encompasses every aspect of recovery and focuses on long-term results. The frameworks and tools in this book are all geared towards an approach that calms the nervous systems, reconditions your brain and body appropriately, and helps you build your capacity so you can live a normal life again. You can brain retrain til the cows come home, but if you're pushing and crashing no one technique will fix that. These processes and frameworks retrain your brain and body so as you read along and participate appropriately, change can occur.

I often say that you can't heal in the same environment you got sick in. Your inner and outer environments need to be assessed and upgraded.

~~~~~~

**Remember, you are a multi-dimensional
human being so having a holistic
and multi-dimensional approach is
the key to long-term success.**

~~~~~~

I was lucky in the fact that I knew recovery was possible because a famous footballer called Alastair Lynch suffered from CFS and recovered. He even wrote a book about his journey and said that beating CFS was his greatest achievement. After seeing Alastair recover I knew I could too. Before I discovered Alastair's story, the greatest hope I was given was "to manage the condition."

I even went to a support group for help, but when I got there I felt worse. It was a bunch of people sitting in a circle discussing their symptoms. No one mentioned getting better. I felt super depressed after that because I wanted to discuss how we could band together and get better. I swore I would never return to a group like that again. And I invite you to do the same, if you want to get better, stop being in circles and environments that bring you down. Of course if it's helpful and useful, keep doing it!

I am so grateful that Alastair shared his story, otherwise maybe that seed of hope may not have germinated in my psyche. With CFS, you get so bombarded with messages that you can't get better, that there is no cure, that it can become too scary to believe otherwise. It's easier to shut yourself off from the possibility of being healthy and living again than being disappointed for the rest of your life. Again this is not your fault. You have been let down by the medical system.

Having an illness like CFS is hard enough as it is, managing it for the rest of your life is a full time job, and not a fun one. But it doesn't have to be a matter of managing it, you can overcome it altogether. And yes, recovery is holistic, and yes recovery is starting where you are - but recovery is possible. It happens all the time.

I found recovering challenging because I was fixated on having the old me back and instead of building the new me. I had to build a whole new foundation from zero. But foundations start at ground-zero, and get built from there.

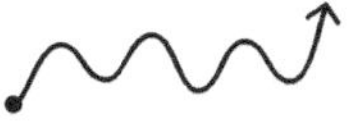

I'm a huge advocate for taking a holistic approach to CFS because:

1. It works
2. You're not a robot.

You are a multi-faceted human being and each day will be different depending on how you sleep, what you eat, your daily stress levels and what you have done the previous day/s before.

When it comes to symptom management and pacing yourself, and doing things like graded exercise therapy; the problem is these processes are inflexible in nature and can be incorrectly prescribed and can be detrimental to your health and recovery. It can either keep you stuck or pull you backwards. **It does not take into account that each day will be different and you're not programmable like a robot. A fixed, inflexible approach can keep you stuck for years.**

Taking a holistic approach helps you stabilize your health in a way that focuses on wellbeing not symptoms, on building your personal capacity rather than measuring you against a system. Body wisdom and knowing what is right for you is the very first step. More on this later.

Making progress is an important part of your recovery and that progress needs to be sustainable and enjoyable. That's how you get your life back!

In saying that there are many myths that still get a lot of attention. Let me address the most common three.

MYTHBUSTING

Myth 1 - Pacing yourself will return your health

I do not believe that pacing is the answer—I believe that baseline is the answer, and there's a huge difference. (Don't worry, baseline is coming up in chapter 6, so get excited).

Pacing is where you are given a fixed, structured routine and you cannot deviate from that routine, no matter what.

Pacing teaches you to track symptoms and to focus on a fixed,restricted plan. Now this can be useful initially, especially if it helps you stop overdoing it, but it can keep you stuck for years as you will stay at that lower level and never know how or when to progress.

On the other hand, pacing can make you go backwards if you are on a fixed plan. So many doctors or physiotherapists who don't fully understand CFS, often overprescribe activity to patients which leaves them feeling worse. Usually blanket comments like, "walk for ten minutes a day," or "just get outside," can be detrimental. Because one; it is probably too much for that person's current capacity. And two; the patient believes they have to do it every day and to stick to it exactly (which isn't smart if the person has had poor sleep or ongoing stress). Activity needs to have a flexible approach based on the key factors in recovery, which you will learn in the next chapter.

In contrast, baseline is being able to have a flexible routine and structure that allows you to do what you can without feeling worse in any given moment.

Forming a baseline and eventually tuning into your body (not symptoms) is the ultimate goal. When you master your baseline, you can start to understand exactly what to do and when to do it based on how you feel. And when you do that, it allows more freedom and greater capacity to be built over time, which will then help you start living again.

This is *body wisdom*.

All of this will help you have more consistency. And the body and brain love consistency. Why? Because they can adapt to it over time. This is how progress happens.

Are you excited for the next chapter already? I hope so.

Myth 2 - Following a fixed exercise prescription will return your strength

The second problem I see with specific recovery models is the term "graded exercise therapy" (G.E.T). There are a lot of myths around exercise and movement when it comes to chronic fatigue syndrome and other associated chronic illnesses. With graded exercise therapy, it is a fixed approach and unfortunately it is usually wrongly prescribed in the world of ME/CFS. When it comes to G.E.T, what happens is that people will go to a physiotherapist who will put them through some tests. And then based on those tests, they'll be given an exercise routine; however, this person might not actually be ready for exercise at all. And so, the program that has been given to them has over-prescribed exercise and the client either can't perform it safely or pushes themselves to do it even though their body is screaming a hard no. We tackle this more deeply in chapter 9, Movement.

Myth 3 - Tackling one symptom at a time will eventually heal the CFS

The problem most people face when trying to recover on their own is having a symptom-focused approach versus a health-focused one. They're busy going down the symptoms rabbit hole, trying to find cures for one symptom at a time rather than looking at the holistic picture. They spend their time finding solutions for their leg pain or their headaches, dizziness or gut irritability. With a quick few keywords into Dr. Google, forty tabs open with a slew of opinions, quick fix pills, special diets (we've all been there) and gadgets that promise to work. You try them all hoping one of them will stick, only to find out that none of them work.

Have you ever noticed when you focus on trying to fix or get rid of your symptoms, your symptoms get worse? This is what happens to all the clients we work with around the world. Up until they join our recovery program, they have been chasing symptoms and getting nowhere. As soon as they embark on a holistic health-focused approach and play the long game to recovery, guess what? Their health starts to improve.

Now I'm not saying don't do or use things that can help calm your nervous system and create more ease for yourself, but when the focus is on trying to fix your symptoms in the hope that your CFS will go away, you're going to come up short and disappointed every time. The anxiety alone from fixating on your symptoms can exacerbate your symptoms. It's a vicious cycle to fall into and one that won't help you in the long term with getting healthy and starting to live again.

A SIMPLE SUM

I know this may sound oversimplified in this complicated mine-field of CFS but I have one big health gauge that I focus on. People often ask me if the CFS Health program will treat their illness and fix their symptoms. My reply is no. *(Cue background gasps of shock).*

It sounds astonishing but it's true. We don't actually treat the illness. Instead, we have a health-solution approach that treats the individual on becoming healthy again, as you get healthier, your symptoms naturally go down.

As a result of the holistic program, your immune system improves, your brain and gut health improves (hello healthy poos), your nervous system regulates appropriately, your sleep and circadian rhythm get back in sync, your mood gets better and everything else starts to feel better too. And when that happens, symptoms start to dissipate over time and your health goes up.

So the simple health sum is = health goes up, symptoms go down.

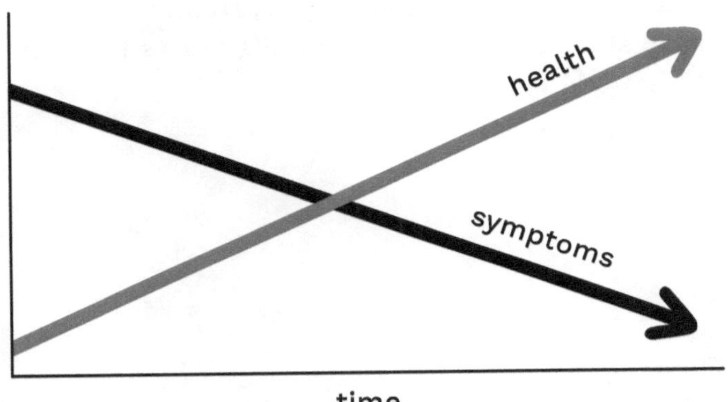

TAKEAWAYS

RECOVERY IS BROKEN DOWN INTO THREE STAGES: Restore, Re-strengthen, and Re-integration. Each stage requires a different energy output and approach. Each stage is unique to you.

STAGE 1—RESTORE: In the acute phase, the focus is on conserving energy, not exercising or pushing beyond capacity. Mistakes in this stage can worsen symptoms, and pushing too hard leads to a cycle of crashing.

STAGE 2—RE-STRENGTHEN: This phase marks the start of rebuilding energy. Gradual, structured activities should be introduced based on the body's increasing ability to handle energy output without causing crashes.

STAGE 3—RE-INTEGRATION: In the final stage, individuals begin to reintegrate into normal life, using lessons from earlier stages. The body adapts to higher energy outputs, and individuals can shift between energy zones (rest, light energy output and high energy output). As you get stronger and healthier your body can adapt appropriately to more stimulus over time. Here energy creates energy. This is the sexy stage of recovery where life starts to open up.

HOLISTIC APPROACH. Recovery isn't just physical but also mental and emotional. Tailoring nutrition, sleep, mindset, and movement to the recovery stage is crucial, avoiding pushing too hard or focusing solely on symptoms. Focusing on improving overall health rather than chasing symptom relief is more effective. As health goes up, symptoms go down.

RECOVERY INSPIRATION

Time to get your recovery journey underway with a free training.

Download our free training about the Three Stage Recovery Framework and learn what to avoid so you don't have to keep going around in circles with "quick fixes."

CHAPTER 5

Energy and You

ENERGY CREDITS

When we talk about "energy" in the context of chronic fatigue syndrome, we're not just talking about the get-up-and-go kind. We're talking about the deep, cellular fuel that your body uses to function—physically, emotionally and mentally. It's the currency your body spends on everything from digesting food to standing up, to processing emotions, to socializing and having a conversation, to basic movement and functioning.

A helpful way to think about energy is in the form of "energy credits." Some days you might have ten energy credits, and other days you might only have two to spend. Every activity costs something—making a meal, going to the bathroom, texting a friend, scrolling your phone, walking, and other activities. Even thoughts and emotions cost energy.

The problem most people with CFS run into is that they're constantly spending more credits than they have in the energy bank. And just like with money, when you overspend energy, you go into debt. Being in debt is never fun; being in energy debt is no different—and that's when crashes happen. You feel foggy, heavy, exhausted, and sometimes even worse than you did before. This is why having a baseline plan specific to you and where you're at is vital for recovery.

You've probably heard the phrase, "You can't pour from an empty cup." It's not just a nice idea—it's a biological truth. You can't keep giving, doing, pushing, or showing up if your cup is empty. Recovery is about learning how to fill your cup first (or at least equal if you have kids) and then protecting it. Why? Because your future self and people around you will thank you for it.

That might mean saying no, resting before you're exhausted, or choosing the quiet option over the busy one.

Remember, health *first* is the option you want to choose here. The goal isn't to do nothing with your energy, but to spend it wisely—on things that matter, that uplift you, and that don't leave you drained.

Energy is your most precious resource right now. Start treating it that way and you'll start to notice something powerful: energy generates energy. The more you protect and replenish it, the more it grows.

Don't Wait for Energy to Return
Before Starting Recovery

I used to believe that I had to wait for energy to come before I could start my recovery. But it never came. It wasn't until I shifted my focus from waiting for energy to come to focusing on building my strength, stamina and capacity that my energy started to return.

Once I got better and started helping others recover, I started to notice the same theme. People were getting sent to me from all over the world through word-of-mouth, and most of them had been told by their doctors to just rest and wait until they got better. The problem was that after 6–12 months of laying around waiting to get better, they got worse. It was like their bodies were starting to rot away, they became more deconditioned, their sleep got worse, their immune system weakened and overall they just felt no different, or worse.

When they started following the program, they too realized that it wasn't about waiting for energy to come but rather building strength and capacity in their brains and bodies so they could do more without feeling worse. (We take a deep dive into this throughout the next chapter.)

The entire body and brain's energy system is affected when experiencing chronic fatigue syndrome (e.g., central nervous system, hormonal system, circadian rhythm). The energy is either being poorly distributed (unregulated systems) and/or the energy that is available is being used to help your body heal. From a subjective viewpoint, purely from observing my clients and going through it myself, it is almost always the case that energy is the last thing to come back online when it comes to recovery from ME/CFS, and it usually starts to return in the middle to later stages of recovery.

From a scientific point of view, there are several potential reasons why energy may be slow to return to people recovering from CFS. One possibility is that the condition itself may cause long-lasting changes in the body's energy systems, such as altered metabolism or mitochondrial dysfunction (mitochondrial membranes are responsible for generating energy for a cell). The experience of prolonged fatigue may lead to changes in the way the brain processes information and regulates energy levels. These changes may take time to fully reverse, even after the underlying cause of the CFS has been addressed.

It is so important to focus on building health, capacity and stamina. By doing that, you are restoring health in your system appropriately and therefore all systems will function better, which means better energy usage and efficiency and better energy output.

The bottom line: **do not wait for energy to come in order to start your recovery.**

Energy will come as you start to get better, and as hard as it is, you have to be patient. (Handy hint, the next chapter spells out how to do this).

The "Working in and Working Out" Philosophy

Many years ago, a holistic health practitioner called Paul Chek in the United States introduced me to a philosophy that he called "working in and working out." It struck me as a helpful way to approach our overall energy levels from a day-to-day, week-to-week and even month-to-month outlook.

Essentially, there are energy "in" activities that bring us energy, and then there are energy "out" activities that deplete energy.

Energy in = restores energy

Energy out = expends energy

Neither are good or bad. They just are, and it's important to know what is right and appropriate for you at each stage of your recovery.

"Energy out" activities don't have to be bad though, and in fact they can be things that bring you immense joy. Over time as you start the recovery process, you need to make sure there are "energy out" activities in your daily routine so that you can exert enough energy appropriately so by the end of the day you are "good tired," which helps you sleep better at night.

Of course, if you're in the beginning stages (like stage 1), the "energy out" activities are going to be on the smaller side to start with, as your capacity is reduced already and there aren't excess reserves to use, so we don't want to deplete you any more than you need. Don't worry, this will get better over time as you start to build your baseline.

As you move through the stages and increase your capacity, you will start to do more "energy out" activities. In fact, as you progress, you'll find that energy creates more energy. What once drained you in stage 1, now energizes you in stage 3. For example, spending time with friends takes energy, but it can also make you feel energized. The same goes for doing yoga or gardening.

One of the key areas we want to look at when it comes to your energy is energy drainers. We certainly don't need an extra dose of these. Now I know that many things can drain your energy, not to mention some people can too. But I've noticed some common themes that can really rob your charge.

ENERGY DRAINERS
Your attitude

Every thought you have sets the tone for how you feel. Yep. Your attitude to life can be a real drainer if you don't take control of it. Negative thought patterns suck the little energy you have left. If you wake up, look outside and say, "Oh, that's another cloudy day. What a crappy day." Then you're already responding as if you're not in control of how you feel. It's as if it's the weather's fault for making you feel bad. Instead, re-route your thinking, and your brain will start to believe you. For example, instead of moaning about the weather, think about how nice it is to be tucked inside and warm on a rainy day. It sounds so simple, but sometimes simplicity works best. We can't always control our circumstances, but we can certainly use our attitude in a way that serves us.

Doomscrolling

It's time to call out the elephant in the room—researching negative information online—also known as "doomscrolling." When you have a problem like CFS, it's easy to do, right? You jump on Google, you type in your problem, and then all of a sudden, countless things pop up and you start to freak out. Mostly, it just compounds the exhaustion and increases stress and confusion. And yes, it can be useful sometimes, but most of the time it's not. So, the next time you catch yourself deep into the rabbit hole, ask yourself: *Is what I'm doing right now serving me or my future self, and is it useful?* I am confident that the answer is almost always no.

Comparison

A common saying is, "Comparison is the thief of joy." And it's true. Comparison robs us of our precious energy every single day. It can send you into a downward spiral. Comparing yourself to other people is a waste of time because you don't know what anyone else is going through. Most of us present our best selves to the world. Social media is saturated with manufactured lives. It is an entire online world designed for comments and likes and comparisons. The only person you can control is yourself. Start to focus on that, and stop comparing yourself to your past self, or where you're at right now, or somebody else. Don't compare your chapter one with someone's chapter twenty. Instead, focus on what you can do today. That'll free up a lot of energy and it will elevate your joy levels.

People-pleasing and perfectionism

Can the people pleasers and perfectionists in the room raise your hand? It's very common for people with CFS to have traits of people-pleasing and perfectionism. 90% of the clients we work with have some form of people-pleasing or perfectionism traits. We dive into this in chapter 7 on Mindset.

Have you ever noticed how draining it is to try and be nice and happy all the time? Have you ever noticed how exhausting it is to over-give, and not receive much back?

Have you ever noticed that because you over-give, people expect you to overgive a lot and then you feel like you're being taken for granted?

The people-pleaser inside of you is making you more exhausted than you realize. But often there's something deeper lurking underneath the people-pleasing actions. Some inner beliefs like, *I'm not enough, I'm not worthy*; or the constant need to prove yourself in order to be loved.

The most loving thing you can do is stop trying to please everyone and take care of yourself properly. People will respect you and you will reap the benefits in "energy credits" too. You will be empowered, instead of feeling trampled on.

The same rules apply for perfectionism. Imagine trying to be perfect all the time? How exhausting. Look behind the reasons you are trying to be perfect and address the root cause. Once you do this, perfectionism can lessen and energy credits will return. Not to mention life will become more fun and less serious. CFS is serious enough, you don't need more of it. You need less of it.

Your bedroom

CFS and bedrooms! What can I say? Sufferers know that when you're in your bedroom all day, every day, it can create a massive energy downfall. Our bedrooms are associated with sleep. And of course, sleep is vital, and we need it, but if we're in our bedrooms all the time—in a darkened room, with not much air—it can be quite draining without you even realizing. I recommend trying to get out of the bedroom and into the lounge room at least. Even better if you can make it outside and get some fresh air. If your bedroom is where you spend most of your time, then brighten it up and make sure it's full of light and fresh air. Surround yourself with things that bring you joy—it could be fresh flowers, photos that make you happy, your own vision board with words and images depicting your future life. That way you can continue to dream while you work towards your recovery.

Dehydration

I know this sounds simple, but you'd be surprised how often simple things are overlooked. Dehydration can be a superdrainer! It's really important to drink enough water (between 1.5–2 liters per day). Even 5% or 10% dehydration can cause a massive lack of energy in your body. Hydrate that incredible body of yours and you will reap the benefits.

Television

Public confession—I don't have a TV in my house. I like to sit in peace and quiet rather than watch shows that demotivate me, are uninspiring, and are mostly negative. But many people like TV, and if you're one of them—then I suggest watching shows and movies that are positive, uplifting and inspiring. It can be non-fiction or fiction, but the important thing is to make sure you're not watching it to mindlessly fill your day. Instead, choose carefully and purposefully what you consume.

The internet

Obviously the internet is fantastic because it connects us to things that we need; however, sitting on the internet doing passive tasks can actually be quite draining. It will suck your energy faster than you can say "www." It doesn't mean that you've got to stop searching and enjoying exploring and surfing the net, it means being smarter with how much time you spend on it. Like television, make sure the content you are consuming or tasks you are doing are purposeful and life enhancing. One of the things you'll find is once you stop doing all the things that create noise in your life, you start to bring back peace, harmony and centeredness. As a result, you'll have more energy to do things you love.

Social media

Nowadays, we've got two lives. We've got our physical life and then we've got an online life. We need to combine them and ask ourselves: *Am I living my life the way I would love to? Is being online all the time and having that identity helping me?*

To put it plainly, social media is an addiction. I know a lot of people struggle with it and that includes myself. It's something that we all must be aware of and question if it's inspiring us or draining us? This may mean cutting back on the hours we use it or being intentional with the content we consume and the people we follow or interact with. From time to time, to increase focus and presence in my life, I delete social media off my phone for certain hours. Let's say I want to wake up and use my day intentionally, I delete social media apps off my phone the night before, so when I wake up there is zero chance for distraction. Then at a certain time the next day, let's say the afternoon, I re-install it if I want to use it again.

Intentional choices are key.

Clothing

This may sound random and I'm not one for giving fashion advice, but I swear this is a game-changer. I'd like you to try this at home. Change into "daytime" and "nighttime" clothes. Sounds a bit strange, doesn't it? I tell many of my clients who are housebound, to change out of their pajamas into their normal daily clothes, even if they are not leaving the house. The brain associates pajamas with sleep and we don't want the brain associating pajamas with sleep all day. If you don't get changed out of your pajamas and into "day" clothes, it creates this kind of depressed, sluggish feeling. Changing into something like jeans and a sweater is a way to signal to your brain that you're awake, you're doing things, and you're living your life. The switching out of your sleepwear and into your daytime clothes will actually help you with your sleep if you stick to it. It will help you feel more awake during the day compared to lounging in your pajamas all day. There's research that backs up how "dopamine dressing" can enhance your mood. Now I'm not talking about sitting around in your best cocktail dress all day, but I mean wearing clothes that make you feel happy. Teaching your brain that there is a big difference between night and day. Give it a go!

Little by little becomes a lot

Consistency over intensity is really the key to success. You might think that some of these changes are so small that they seem insignificant. But the truth is little by little becomes a lot, and making small consistent changes in your everyday life over time will eventually lead you to recovery.

LET'S SAY THE F WORD

Now, sometimes in life we are forced to drop an f-bomb or two! And there's one f-word that CFS sufferers can't avoid, and that is *fatigue*. It's the crippling phenomenon we find hard to explain to others and even understand ourselves.

It's important to know that there are six types of fatigue that result from chronic fatigue syndrome. We are going to identify them and then take steps to combat them. Yes, knowledge is power.

Social Fatigue

This often goes unnoticed. I have a lot of clients who go to an event, a wedding, an engagement party, a birthday party, or even just a cup of tea with one close friend and they're exhausted afterwards, and they don't know why.

They say, "I was literally only talking. How can I be so tired from that?"

Yes, but there's a cognitive load that happens when interacting with people. Particularly if you are at a low capacity, or your brain and body are simply not used to the stimulus of socializing anymore. It's best to make sure you start to incrementally socialize; appropriately for where you're at in your capacity. For example, starting with short phone calls or even voice messages and then eventually home visits before graduating to hour-long outings and bigger events. Of course, there will be major events like weddings and birthday parties that you don't want to miss out on, so setting strategies in place to conserve your energy can be useful. This could include stepping away every hour or so and sitting in a quiet space (if possible) or finding someone you're comfortable to sit in silence with. Doing some form of "energy in" activities to cultivate calm and restoration will help massively. Over time, it will get better, and you will start to be able to handle and adapt to those types of situations a lot better.

Emotional Fatigue

Emotional fatigue ties into social fatigue but it's a little different. Emotional fatigue is when you've been under emotional pressure. There are two types:

1. From self—putting too much pressure on yourself, and your perfectionistic thinking is stressing you out like crazy.

2. From others—interpersonal relationships, potentially strained friendships, particularly when you're going through something like chronic illness.

It is common to lose friends because a lot of people don't understand what you're going through. They might think that you're making it up, that you are not a good friend, that you don't care about them. The truth is different. You would love to be able to hang out with your friends and enjoy your time, but you simply can't right now. You're doing the best you can to navigate a very challenging time.

So emotional fatigue is the emotional burden you feel and experience when you feel out of control.

Boundaries also play an important role (or the violation of boundaries). If you're not good at setting boundaries, or are a chronic people-pleaser, you'll find that you will often get walked over by others, and then emotional fatigue will be a factor.

We look at emotional fatigue like a leaky bucket. If your bucket is sealed, then everything's fine. But if there's holes in the bucket, let's say you're not good at boundaries and you keep saying yes to things you want to say no to, then you're going to be emotionally fatigued. Your energy will drain quicker than you can say "empty bucket." It's important to check in with yourself, assess your boundaries, and ask yourself if you're honoring where you're at in your emotional capacity? If you find this pattern cycles, then work with a coach or an online recovery program like ours that teaches you the skill of setting healthy boundaries. Boundaries can be an act of self-love. I cover this in more depth in chapter 7 on Mindset.

Physical Fatigue

This is the one we're all most familiar with, the physical activities. Your daily activity is vital to your wellbeing. Having the correct baseline for 'energy in' and 'energy out' is the most important part to building your physical capacity. Having a correct baseline means that you can do things without feeling any worse than you currently do. When you do that, you start to build repetition, you start to build consistency, and your brain and body start to adapt appropriately to the stimulus you give it. If you are experiencing physical fatigue, it could be that you're overdoing it for where you are currently at. It's a big one, and a lot of people don't even realize they're doing it. It's the push-crash cycle that is so common. Stay tuned for more on this in the next chapter.

Hormonal Fatigue

Hormonal fatigue applies to both men and women, but it particularly affects people who menstruate. There are four stages of the menstruation cycle: menstruation, follicular phase, ovulation and the luteal phase. Only one of the four stages has positive symptoms and that's the follicular phase, whereas the other three, and in particular menstruation and the luteal phase, often comes with mood swings, stress, sadness, and fatigue. Even a healthy person will have a noticeable difference in their energy levels and will need to adjust their lifestyle to match (i.e., eating more calories and doing less intense activities or exercise). This fatigue will obviously affect a person with CFS even more, so it's extremely important to be aware of the effects of the menstruation cycle and adjust accordingly.

We have specific training in our mentorship recovery program, all about women's hormonal health and in that training, we teach you how to maneuver your baseline around your cycle so that you can adapt appropriately. The common problem I see is that people keep trying to stick to the same routine and structure every single week. But menstruation can play a key factor in women's health and adapting to it is important. Menstruation matters.

Cognitive Fatigue

Cognition is the output of energy using our brain. This can be anything from reading, watching TV or videos on the internet, working, studying, or even the mental load of deciding what to have for dinner this week. When we engage with too much content, we can go too far and turn a "good" mental tiredness into a cognitive overload that makes even thinking about a decision too difficult. For example, we've had members who enroll in the program, and they watch every video we have available straight away and overwhelm themselves.

You might catch yourself at home doing that too, where it's something you really want to learn or you want to devour hours of something, and then halfway through your brain is like, "Ah, no, I can't do this anymore." And that's where we need to give ourselves a cognitive break. Cognitive overload is a real thing, and we need to make sure that we're not doing that. Even when you're healthy, it's important that you don't cognitively overload yourself and be too content-heavy.

Spiritual Fatigue

This is not specifically about religion (though it can be), but more so an identity crisis. You're in a chasm between what you don't want and what you want, and it can feel like there's a gap between your old self, your present self, and your future self.

Common phrases are:

"I don't know what I want to do with my life."

"This sucks. I don't want to keep feeling this way, but how will I create the new life that I want?"

"I just want my old life back."

"I don't know who I am anymore."

This is why I have developed an up-level part in our program, called lifestyle integration, so people can design and create a life that they want. You may not want to go back to the old life that possibly got you sick in the first place (with burnout or unhealthy habits), but you want to create a life that is healthy and aligned with the type of person you want to be now and into the future. Spiritual fatigue starts to go away as you start to integrate into the life that you want.

Why This Matters

As you can see, all these different types of fatigue can affect you at any time. It's important to be able to recognize it so that you can modify your behaviors and reduce the burden of fatigue. It's also important so that you can approach your recovery from a calm and controlled state. If you approach recovery in a desperate and overwhelmed state where you are looking for a supplement or quick fix, then you will cancel out any benefit those fixes would have.

I want to invite you to completely change your approach. I want you to give yourself a break from the types of fatigue you *can* control, which is social, emotional, cognitive and spiritual. Work on your daily habits to get rid of energy drainers and create a sense of calmness and peace. This approach is the primer for recovery. It's the same as painting a house— you must sand back the walls and then do the priming coat before adding the actual paint. Sure, going straight on with the paint would add the color, but it will be flaky, uneven and not stick right in certain places. It certainly won't last. This is the same approach we need to take with both our mindset and our energy sources when coming into recovery.

ENERGY GAINERS

Now, energy gainers are different for everyone depending on what stage they are in their recovery. Energy gainers are anything that restores calm in the body and brain, settles the nervous system, and has rejuvenating qualities. This can be resting, meditating, gentle movement or whatever nourishes you energetically.

Thinking about your energy gainers and energy drainers can be very helpful. I suggest you draw a line down the middle of a piece of paper and list ten energy gainers and energy drainers. Energy gainers - give you energy. Energy drainers - drain your energy.

Keep this list handy as you focus on your recovery.

List of energy gainers	**List of energy drainers**
1.	1.
2.	2.
3.	3.
4.	4.
5.	5.
6.	6.
7.	7.
8.	8.
9.	9.
10.	10.

FOMO VS JOMO

Okay, we've discussed our Mojo. Now let's talk about FOMO. Yep the Fear Of Missing Out (FOMO). I had a bad case of FOMO when I had CFS. Having chronic fatigue syndrome, can feel like life is passing you by. That you always have to miss out on all the fun stuff.

The suffering and pain that you already have is only amplified when you're invited to an event or hangout and all of a sudden you're torn between risking your health or sitting at home with FOMO. Not great options. It sucks big time.

For me, it was wanting to socialize with friends, run as hard as I possibly could, and just go to damn school to have some fun. It felt like life had trapped me and I couldn't do anything. I was lying in misery thinking, *Why me? Life is unfair.* This went on for years. I had no idea I was creating more suffering by allowing FOMO to take over my days.

It wasn't until I got into acceptance mode, that things got easier. I realized that to get to where I wanted to be, I had to make hard decisions in my life now in order to create the future life I wanted.

As the old saying goes…

Hard decisions = easy life. Easy decisions = hard life.

I had to say no to things that I really wanted to do but weren't good or appropriate for me at the time. Things that would have made me overdo it or go beyond my current capacity. If I wanted to get my life back, I had to stay focused on things that helped me, not hindered me. It wasn't easy, but it was worth it.

**I had to say a million little no's for the
one big yes, which was recovery.
I had to turn moments of FOMO
into JOMO (joy of missing out).**

As I got really focused and disciplined, I started feeling good about what I was doing. I started to notice moments of inner peace and joy I hadn't felt for years.

Of course this started small, but it built up into bigger things over time. As I started to get better, my agency over what I could and couldn't do grew ever bigger. It was such a great, satisfying feeling having confidence in my ability and my growing capacity to do more without going backwards.

I'm sharing this with you because initially it was hard. Going from FOMO to JOMO felt like an almost impossible task. But once I started to truly accept where I was at, I was able to relish in JOMO and saying no to things started to feel good because **I was choosing my recovery instead**. Feeling empowered was helping me heal, and doing the right things at the right time felt good. This is when real tangible progress happened in my recovery.

Signs you are living in FOMO
- You have a lot of jealous feelings.
- You experience unnecessary emotional/mental suffering on top of the pain of CFS.
- You're constantly wishing for your life to be different than it is.
- You say yes regularly even though it doesn't feel right in your body.
- You feel desperate a lot of the time. Like you must catch up on lost time.

Signs you are living in JOMO

- You are feeling more and more content in your life.
- You have accepted where you are at.
- You give yourself more grace and compassion versus hate and self-sabotage.
- You start to enjoy saying no and feel good about your decision.
- You start to see and feel glimmers of hope and a brighter future.

Making the jump from FOMO to JOMO does require courage; however, when you do, you will feel better day-to-day in your decisions and live in a place of healing. Choose joy!

So, who's going to JOMO town with me?

THE POWER OF CALMNESS

This leads straight into why it's important to remain calm and remove stressors. One of the most underestimated and often overlooked factors in chronic fatigue syndrome recovery is calmness. Not just the absence of chaos, but true inner calm—the kind that lets your body take a deep sigh and say, "I'm safe now."

Cortisol and the Stress Loop

When you're under stress—whether it's emotional, physical, or mental—your body releases a hormone called cortisol. It's part of the "fight or flight" response, and in small doses, cortisol is helpful. It gives you a temporary boost of energy, increases alertness, and helps you respond to danger.

But here's the problem: chronic stress means chronic cortisol, and over time, this completely dysregulates your system. High or imbalanced cortisol levels can wreak havoc on your immune function, your sleep, your digestion, your mood, and yes—your energy levels.

The whole goal is to move out of the sympathetic nervous system and move into the parasympathetic nervous system where calm lives. Initially, we need to bring calmness back into the body so you can stabilize and then progress.

Think of it this way: cortisol is a short-term emergency tool. It's not designed to be your body's daily operating system, but for many people with CFS, it's like the stress switch got flipped on one day and never got turned back off. This constant state of activation is exhausting. Your body doesn't have the chance to get into the "rest and repair" mode that it needs in order to heal and it gets compounded by the desperation to get better. When we stress out about which fix to try, which program to enroll in, what supplements to take or what diet to try, we end up pushing these cortisol levels higher and doing more damage.

Calm Is Not a Luxury—It's a Requirement

Modern society has conditioned us to believe that rest or calmness is something we *earn* after we've done all the hard work and that if we have too much, then we're lazy or unmotivated.

However, this is a very Western ideal and Eastern cultures value calmness and peace much more, hence why meditation and yoga come from those parts of the world. When healing from CFS, we need to scrap the idea that being calm or at peace has to be earned and instead embed it into our everyday lives.

Remember, chronic fatigue syndrome does not affect lazy people. You are not lazy for resting, you are resting when you need to, so you get healthy.

***

Calmness *is* the hard work.
It's the thing that makes all the
other healing possible.

***

We need to flip the script on what healing looks like. It's not always supplements and protocols and to-do lists. Often, it looks like doing less. Saying no. Slowing down. Choosing softness over urgency. When you bring more calm into your life—consistently, not just occasionally—you send your body a powerful message: you are safe. And safety is the first prerequisite for healing.

When your nervous system is calm, a whole cascade of positive things happens inside your body:

- Your parasympathetic nervous system (the "rest and digest" system) kicks in.
- Your heart rate slows down and your blood pressure stabilizes.

- Your digestive system functions better (which means you absorb more nutrients).
- Your immune system becomes more balanced and less inflammatory.
- Your sleep improves (deep, restorative sleep is essential for energy repair).
- Your hormones start to rebalance.
- Your brain fog begins to clear.

All of this adds up to one thing: energy restoration. True, cellular energy. Not caffeine energy or adrenaline energy, but real vitality.

Stress Isn't Just in Your Head

It's important to note that stress doesn't always look like worry or anxiety. Sometimes it's subtle. Sometimes it's a constant mental to-do list running in the background, perfectionism, or a sense of guilt for not being "productive." Sometimes it's physical—like being in a noisy environment or eating food that doesn't agree with you. Sometimes it's emotional—feeling unseen, unsupported, or disconnected.

Even good things can be stressful if your nervous system isn't ready for them. A long phone call with a loved one, a short walk around the block, a social gathering—they might bring joy, but they still take energy. And that's okay. It means we need to be gentle and aware of our own capacity.

Stress can also come from internal dialogue. That voice that says, *You should be better by now,* or *You're not doing enough.* That inner critic might seem like it's motivating you, but it's actually pushing your stress hormones up and your energy down. Take it easy on yourself.

Practical Ways to Invite Calm In

So how do you actually cultivate calmness when life feels overwhelming, and your body is constantly tired? Start small. Consistency is more important than intensity. Here are a few gentle, calming practices you can try:

Slow breathing: Inhale for 4 counts, exhale for 6. Do this for two minutes. This signals to your brain that it's okay to relax.

Progressive muscle relaxation: Tense and release each muscle group in your body, from head to toe.

Grounding exercises: Sit with your feet flat on the ground, close your eyes, and feel the weight of your body being supported.

Nature time: Even a few minutes outside—listening to birds, feeling the sun, or touching a tree—can calm the nervous system.

Digital boundaries: Limit your time on screens, especially in the morning and evening. This helps reduce mental overstimulation.

Affirmations or calming mantras: Repeating phrases like "I am safe," "I trust the process," or "My body knows how to heal" can quiet your inner critic and soothe your nervous system.

Calm spaces: Create a little sanctuary in your home that is designated for mindful resting. Think cozy blankets, soft lighting, soothing scents, or whatever makes you feel most at ease.

Non-sleep deep rest (yoga nidra): Another wonderful way to calm the nervous system.

**Calm supports our nervous systems;
it's like a constant dialogue reassuring
our body that it is safe.**

TAKEAWAYS

ALL THINGS ENERGY: Energy is the currency of your body, and it's used on everything from digesting food to standing up and having a conversation. People with CFS have a much lower amount of energy than their healthy selves, making it difficult to adapt to this new level. During recovery, it's important to never overspend on energy, not to wait for energy to return before starting recovery and to have a balance between "energy in" and "energy out" activities. It's also integral to ditch any "energy drainers" and invest in "energy gainers."

THE DIFFERENT TYPES OF FATIGUE: There are six types of fatigue: social, emotional, physical, hormonal, cognitive, and spiritual. All can be drained by CFS and it's helpful to break them down and understand what they are so you know how to monitor and build each one back up.

CHOOSE JOMO: Having CFS means saying no a lot, and this can mean there's a lot of guilt and FOMO about missing events. However, when we shift our mindset and allow ourselves to put our recovery first, we can find the joy in missing out (JOMO).

INVITING CALM: The stress hormone, cortisol, is very damaging to our systems when it comes in high doses and for prolonged periods. Therefore, it's far more beneficial for your recovery if you approach it from a place of calm (it's hard, I know) and not burn your energy stressing about achieving certain that are not appropriate for you right now.

RECOVERY INSPIRATION

Download our free e-book to learn how to overcome symptoms once and for all.

CHAPTER 6

It's All About the Baseline

STOP THE CYCLE OF PUSHING AND CRASHING

Have you ever been on a seesaw? When a person sits on each end of a balanced plank, and when one end goes up, the other goes down. Now think of when a person puts all their weight on to their side of the seesaw…it raises you up really high which can feel fun, but as soon as they jump off their side of the seesaw—you come dropping down really fast! It's not much fun on the way down and can actually hurt a lot.

This is just like the push-crash cycle with chronic fatigue syndrome. When you push yourself (and it can feel kind of fun), but the sudden coming down is horrible. You get a short-term high and a long-term low. This often flares your symptoms for days, and even weeks, if you go way too high or too hard.

Like most, when I had CFS I experienced severe pushing and crashing. Early on it was extreme, because I was trying to live up to my old life energy levels and I had little clue what was wrong with me. I'd rest and rest and rest, and then as soon as I had energy to burn, I burnt it all, plus extra. I'd play one game of sport and be totally spent that I'd end up in bed and in pain for the entire week. Sometimes I'd see friends, or go to a party, only to leave halfway through and be totally wiped-out days after. It was a vicious cycle. The chronic ride of push-and-crash made me depressed; I almost gave up on life at one point. It was dark. I was sick and tired of being sick and tired.

Back then, I didn't know anything about my baseline. In fact, to me 'baseline' was a basketball term that represented the white line behind the backboard and hoop. I didn't realize it had anything to do with my health.

It was Dr. Lionel Lubitz, who first gave me the initial understanding of baseline many years ago when he was treating me. I have since added new layers to the baseline framework to help clients build a strong foundation for recovery. One of the things that Dr. Lubitz used to repeat all the time is "you don't want to do too much, but you don't want to do too little." You want to find "your sweet spot."

Finding your baseline is about finding your sweet spot. It's the art of stopping the push-crash cycle and beginning to make progress that lasts. It is about harnessing the energy you have to create more energy over time. Sounds like a dream come true, right? Well, it can be.

Learning about your baseline gives your health **stability.** And, when was the last time your health was stable?

Stopping the extremes of the push-crash cycle brings more order to your daily life and peace to your health, your nervous system and ultimately helps you get back to living normal life over the long term.

Having CFS can feel like being robbed of life, when a sudden burst of energy does spontaneously arise, it's easy to fall into the trap of trying to do everything while this magical energy lasts. And while it can feel good, or you can believe you're fine—often, hours or days later, you come crashing down as you've spent a week's worth of energy credits in one day. It's demoralizing and soul-crushing.

You crash below your baseline and are suddenly thrust into what I call the valley-of-death red zone (sorry for the harsh label but it really feels that shit). This zone is where the onset of symptoms rage and it can feel like you're dying—excruciating pain and symptoms hammer you day and night.

Avoiding the valley-of-death red zone is a great option, because it's very hard to move forward with your recovery if there's no consistency. Remember, your brain and body love consistency. And let's face it, it's very hard to do anything consistently when you feel stuck in the valley-of-death. The only thing you hope to do is survive.

YOUR BASELINE IS YOUR STABILIZATION POINT FOR RECOVERY

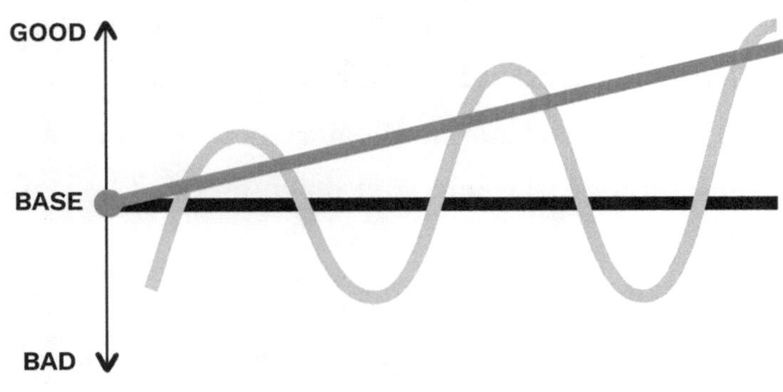

**Your baseline isn't about feeling good all
the time or having heaps of energy;
it's about finding your stabilization
point and sticking to it.**

The problem most people have is they put intensity before consistency, but intensity can't happen until consistency is established. Consistency is key. Consistency will bring you the stability you crave and the freedom you dream of.

Once you understand the baseline, you can apply it with ease. It will stabilize your health and your life and cease the one-step-forward-and-three-steps-back pattern once and for all.

Baseline is one of the golden rules and frameworks that has helped every single client I have worked with get healthy and start living again.

There is a tendency for people with chronic fatigue syndrome to push themselves, but the problem is that pushing yourself beyond your current capacity means your body can't adapt to the stimulus overload in your system. And because it can't adapt, it throws your autonomic nervous system haywire, and your brain and body go into shut down mode. The result? You crash! Hard.

But here's the brilliant thing—you aren't at the mercy of the intense push-crash cycle; you can calm its wild ways and stabilize instead.

Some people get worried when it comes to finding their baseline initially. They say things like, "Oh my gosh, I'm going to have to do less all the time."

"I'm going to have to stop my life completely."

I totally get their concern, they may still be holding onto their old identities of being constant doers, the all-or-nothing type folks whose value comes from being "busy" and "pushing all the time."

But the more you resist, the more the problems persist. And then people say, "Will I be like this forever?"

Here's the deal, recovery doesn't have to be forever. But it does require you to make changes to your current reality so you can live the life you want in the future. It's short- term pain for long-term gain.

Find Your Baseline

It takes around two to four weeks to find your baseline using our daily tracker data collection sheets inside our Mentorship Recovery Program.

It begins by recording a few key factors that help you determine what's working for you and what's not. You reflect on how you feel physically, mentally, emotionally, spiritually and cognitively after that two to four week period. This allows you to create a routine that is both nourishing and strengthening.

Here's what to track:
- Sleep/wake times
- Mealtimes and frequency
- Energy "in" activities
- Energy "out" activities
- Energy drainers
- Overall general health wellbeing

What we don't track is symptoms, as that isn't helpful for the health-focused approach, and it can also cause a lot of overwhelming feelings. Tracking symptoms would be a full-time job, and you don't need that on top of everything else you're dealing with.

Example baseline tracker

Category	Mon	Tue
Wake time	9am	8:45am
Mealtimes	Breakfast: 10am Lunch: 1:30pm Dinner: 6:30pm Ate toast for breakfast and got a bit tired mid-morning.	B: 10:15am L: 2pm D: 6pm Ate a later lunch and didn't drink much water.
Energy "in" activities / energy gainers	Mindfully make a cup of tea, meditate and sit in the sun for 5 minutes.	Journaled (AM)
Energy "out" activities (positive)	Light stretching in bed, 2-min walk to the mailbox.	Dishes and light stretching in bed.
Energy drainers	Doomscrolled on Tik Tok for two hours before bed.	Stayed up late watching TV.
Sleep time	10pm	11pm
Overall wellbeing	Calm but tired, anxious in PM.	Flat mood, cognitive fog.

Wed	Thu	Fri
10am	9am	9am
B: 10:30am L: 1:30pm D: 6pm Late breakfast as slept in so wasn't really hungry at lunch.	B: 10am L: 1pm D: 6pm I didn't eat or drink enough today. Try better tomorrow.	B: 10am L: 1pm D: 6:30pm Ate better quality food and more consistently today. Feel better.
Sat in the sun for 10 minutes listening to calming music.	Colored in a picture for 20 minutes, meditated for 5 minutes and sat in the sun for 15 minutes.	Deep breath exercise in the AM, drank tea in the sun with no distractions, and journaled.
20-minute walk, folded laundry (sitting down), vacuumed the house and cooked dinner.	Light stretching in bed, 5-minute walk around the block and made bed.	Light stretching in bed, 5-minute walk around the block and made bed.
Felt guilty for sleeping in and tried to make up for it.	Watched "shit" TV for one hour.	N/A
10:15pm	10pm	10pm
Overdid it, exhausted.	Weak but emotionally stable.	Fragile but feeling a tad more energized than yesterday.

Once you've got this 2-week study, you can create the "Imperfect, Perfect Daily Routine." This will be based on those things which made you feel good and what made you feel not so good. It's all about finding that sweet spot. It will also focus on consistency in your daily routine/structure. This includes sleep/wake/rest times, meal frequency times and adequate nutrition, work "in" activities (activities that give us energy/restore us) and work "out" activities (activities that exert energy). We also add in "joy" moments. Things that bring a little bit of joy to your day, no matter how small or insignificant it may feel. This is the secret ingredient to making your day more enjoyable and fun.

The most important thing about the daily routine is that it doesn't have to be perfect. We call it the "Imperfect, Perfect Daily Routine" because it helps form a routine that feels good without being too strict or controlling. We want a relaxed approach here. Holding on too tight can create more stress and anxiety and you don't need that with your recovery.

**Remember, it's not what you do,
but how you do it that matters.**

To make your "Imperfect, Perfect Daily Routine," start by writing a list of what made you feel good and what didn't over your past two weeks. We will use the example baseline tracker to show you.

What made me feel good	What made me feel bad
Waking up at 9am	Staying up late
Light stretching in bed	Watching too much TV or Tik Toks.
Making my bed	Watching TV that was not fulfilling or engaging
Meditating and journaling in the morning	Walking for too long (more than 5 minutes)
Doing a small walk	Sleeping in
Sitting in the sun	Doing too much housework (more than 1-2 small tasks)
Coloring in	
Going to bed at 10pm	

You can already see here how the daily routine is coming together by the "What made me feel good" column. What we will do now is put this into a time slotted routine and add in "joy moments."

Now remember, you are building the initial base for baseline. This isn't forever, this is to get you set up so your health stabilizes. After that, you can progress and do more of the fun things you want to do. We will cover how to progress in the coming chapters.

Example "Imperfect, Perfect Daily Routine"

Time	Activity
9:00am	Wake up slowly, do light stretching in bed
9:15am	Make bed
9:30am	Morning meditation (5 min) and journaling (10–15 min)
10:00am	Eat breakfast mindfully (no screens, savor, slow pace, sit near window if possible)

Time	Activity
10:30am	Sit in the sun for 15 minutes listening to calming music
11:00am	Gentle walk around the block (5 min)
11:15am	Rest on couch with eyes closed for 45 minutes
12:15pm	Prepare lunch and eat mindfully (no screens, savor, slow pace, sit near window if possible)
1:00pm	Coloring in while listening to music (30 min)—*Joy moment.*
1:30pm	Reading for 30 minutes (audiobook or physical book—something calming or inspiring)
2:00pm	Rest/meditation/energy in breathing
3:00pm	Light snack and herbal tea (mindful pause)
3:15pm	Light household task, if energy allows (e.g., fold laundry, water plants)
4:00pm	Five minutes of restorative strength based movement
5:00pm	Rest
5:30pm	Prepare and eat dinner (quiet atmosphere, no screens, enjoy the food slowly)
6:15pm	Gentle wind-down activity (TV, podcast, or quiet hobby—max 1 hr)
7:15pm	Evening reflection / journal (if energy allows)
7:30pm	Begin bedtime wind-down (low lights, calm music, no screens). Have a shower and stretch lightly
8:00pm	Read / listen to audiobook or podcast for minimum 30 minutes
8:30pm	Lie in bed, breathe deeply, and practice gratitude or calming thoughts
9:00pm	Lights out—sleep

How do I know I have found my baseline?

Your baseline is about being able to do what you can do without feeling any worse than you currently do. It's as simple as that, but simple doesn't mean easy.

You know you have found your baseline when:

- You stop pushing and crashing.
- You're able to maintain your daily routine for two to four weeks without feeling any worse than you currently do.
- Your health is maintained, meaning that you're not getting sick with colds and flus every second week.

From an exercise science standpoint, we get taught about progressive overload, which is where you progressively overload your muscles appropriately for where you're at. When you train different muscle groups, delayed onset muscle soreness (or DOMs) kicks in, and then over time, your muscles rest, repair and regrow. Do this consistently and your muscles grow stronger and stronger over time.

For someone with CFS, we need to dial back the progress overload even more because your brain and body doesn't have the same number of energy credits a healthy person does, and so this is why the baseline framework works so well because we don't ever put you in a major energy output deficit. It's more nuanced and flexible than that. Instead, the building blocks are a little slower, but by doing it this way, it's way safer and more effective so your brain and body can adapt appropriately to the stimulus over time. Take Jamie's story as an example.

JAMIE

A client, Jamie, had an initial capacity that was super low. He found watching a video for more than a few minutes hard, he felt physically weak, and anything he did initially felt hard mentally and emotionally.

The key was starting with where he was, being consistent, and realizing that it was going to be a little bit challenging at the start. But as long as he didn't go beyond his physical and mental threshold, he was able to do little things each day that were appropriate for where he was.

Because his baseline was low, he was beating himself up thinking that the small things he did wouldn't make a difference; it wasn't enough to be considered progress. What he didn't know yet was consistency over intensity eventually wins the game. Kinda like the old fable about the tortoise and the hare. The hare starts off sprinting and the tortoise starts off plodding…but eventually the hare burns out and gets tired and the tortoise plods past him to win the race.

Jamie started with small things: watching five minutes of a recovery training video each day, doing little bits of movement around the house, sitting up in bed, moving to a different room when he was up to it, and of course eating breakfast, snacks, lunch and dinner.

He stuck to that for a few months, and his capacity naturally grew. His days became easier and he was able to add more activity both physically and cognitively over time.. As his capacity threshold increased, the progress cycle continued, and he started to get stronger and healthier than before. After about 1.5 years of doing this recovery work, he was able to go back to work and eventually get back to full-time work, socializing, traveling, weight training, and living a full life.

INCREMENTAL STEPS

It's necessary to maintain your current baseline for a minimum period of two to four weeks before starting to progress, which means that you're not feeling any worse than you currently were two weeks ago and you're not getting a cold and flu every second week. You're not going one step forward, three steps back. You are simply maintaining your current baseline for a minimum of two to four weeks, especially at the start of your recovery. For some it will be longer maintenance periods due to life or stress getting in the way and that's okay.

As your health maintains and your baseline has been solid for two to four weeks, provided you feel comfortable doing so, you can start to expand your baseline appropriately, just like Jamie did. You might add in some cognitive activities or physical ones, or you might expand what you're doing for a little bit of a longer duration. Once you do expand your new level, remember it's okay for you to feel a little bit tired afterwards. As long as you're not going backwards, or it affects how you feel for days on end.

There is a period of adaptation where this new level will take a little bit of getting used to and making it your new normal. This is why maintenance weeks and months are so vital because you need to solidify what you're doing day to day week to week. We're creating safety in the brain and body by doing this appropriately. No more going from zero to hero! No more jumping up in progress without solidifying what you're already doing.

Most people go wrong here. They try to progress too fast and end up going backwards all the time and then wonder why they aren't improving. Hopefully this is making sense now!

There will be times when life gets in the way. There'll be circumstances that set back your goals. You might get a cold or a flu, which healthy people do as well. You don't stop doing the work just because life's gotten in the way. This is when you lean in more, and you reach out for help, whether it be friends, family or CFS Health. I believe that progress is maintaining too. I don't want you to think that making progress is the only way to progress. It's super important to understand that. Maintaining where you're at is just as important as progressing. In fact it's vital for recovery.

THE BASICS FOR BASELINE SUCCESS

Less is more is just for the beginning

Starting small and building your way up is the most effective technique. This is true in any aspect of life, so be *kind* to yourself. If you started learning a language, you wouldn't expect to speak full sentences on the first day; if you learned a new sport, you're not competing after one week of training; and if you want to recover, you're not going to be running three-kilometers in the first week—but that doesn't mean you can't do any movement at all, and it certainly doesn't mean you won't ever run again. One of our past members who recovered from CFS ended up running a marathon.

You can listen to his interview here:

I have seen many past members go from barely being able to walk, talk, or do life, to hiking mountains, running fun runs and trail runs, dancing, skiing, participating in sports, and traveling the world. And all without having to experience symptoms or crash again. It all started with a baseline.

Start building your baseline from your initial capacity, stop pushing and crashing every week, and you will eventually be able to start to do more.

Stop red lining

Red lining is a phrase we use at CFS Health that means you're going over your baseline threshold way too much and your body/ brain can't keep up. One of our health coaches at CFS Health often asks a reflective question to our clients who are constantly pushing and crashing and getting nowhere. He asks, "What's the part of you that makes you constantly red line? What's beneath that?" There's usually a reason behind behavior patterns like this and understanding what it is can often be the key for someone to finally stop the pushing and crashing once and for all.

It's usually things like—feeling guilty about not being "productive" and trying to overcompensate for the days they couldn't do much, having people-pleasing tendencies and struggling to set boundaries, not accepting their current baseline, or a lack of awareness about the impact of pushing the body. Coming to terms with your current baseline, accepting it, and forgiving yourself is the first step to stopping the cycle.

Consistency over intensity matters

It will be hard to stick with your baseline at first, particularly on the days you wake up with more energy than you normally do, as there is a natural tendency to overcompensate for the lack of activity you've had. But **consistency is one of the key signposts for recovery and it trumps intensity every day of the week**.

Little pieces of progress add up to a lot, whereas trying to do everything all at once and then not being able to back it up time and time again will *not* improve your situation. For example, if you're trying to improve your walking ability and want to walk 60 minutes a week, doing it all at once might be way beyond your baseline and leave you feeling exhausted for the rest of the week. Even though you achieved your goal, it didn't make you feel good and left you drained. You would be better off doing 10 minutes of walking each day, which would actually equate to 70 minutes of walking a week, and since you're doing less but more consistently, you won't feel worse off and over time, you'll be able to do more. Makes sense, right?

Don't do nothing!

It's also not about doing nothing. A lot of people are told to rest, rest, rest, and do more rest only to find they go backwards even more, largely due to the deconditioning in the body and their diminishing capacity due to lack of activity. It's not about doing nothing, and it's certainly not about pushing your body and mind beyond its means. It's about finding the sweet spot for your current capacity. If you're in stage 1 restore phase, then rest will be a big part of your routine and structure right now, but in the other stages, we want to start building your overall capacity, strength and stamina so you can do more without feeling worse. As your health gradually increases, your symptoms naturally decrease and you will notice this over time.

You can't wait to get better

It's super important to remember that a lot of people think, *I need to wait to feel better to start getting better.* That couldn't be further from the truth. You need to start now with your baseline so you can get better later. Don't wait for energy to come: start now. Focus on improving your strength, stamina, and capacity appropriately. And over time, the energy will come.

Being in tune with your body is very different to constantly searching for symptoms. Being in tune with your body just means asking yourself—*does this feel appropriate for me in this moment?* versus saying, *Oh no, I have a symptom of being sick so I shouldn't do anything.* That's a reactive response.

Remember, baseline is about doing what you can do without feeling any worse than you currently do. It's not about waiting for symptoms to disappear for you to start. It's not about waiting for energy to come for you to start either. If you do that, you will be waiting for a very long time.

It's normal to not feel great at the start

Know that you're not going to feel great initially, no matter where you're starting from. Even people who are at a 5 out of 10 don't feel good when they start doing stuff, simply because they're used to being a 10 out of 10. Therefore, the level that you're starting at doesn't matter, the same model applies for everyone in terms of starting wherever you are. This isn't a case of waiting for symptoms to fully go or to wait until you feel good enough to start building your capacity—instead, stick to the principles we're teaching here and build your capacity appropriately and consistently from where you're starting from. It also doesn't matter how small your efforts are initially, and a slight energy dip each day or after certain activities during the day are absolutely normal and appropriate. Especially if you haven't done much lately. That's okay. What we want to avoid is huge levels of output that make you feel horrible for days/ weeks on end.

THE HIBERNATION THEORY

I once had a client, Phillip, who said, "Why is just being normal so hard for me?"

I knew what he meant. Why did just living a normal daily life seem so out of reach?

I used to ask myself this same question.

But then I heard about the Hibernation Theory and something rang true.

Our resident doctor Olivia Lesslar shares The Hibernation Theory with the story of a bear. She says, when we think of hibernation, the image that often comes to mind is a bear settling in for a long winter, stockpiling on food, and retreating into a cave until the first thaw of spring. But what if hibernation wasn't just for animals? What if your body, in its innate wisdom, is using a similar mechanism to protect itself? To understand this more, we'll explore an intriguing concept that links the biological phenomenon of hibernation to chronic fatigue syndrome (CFS) and how understanding this might hold a key to recovery.

Dr. Lesslar introduces us to the curious lifecycle of the nematode worm. It thrives under ideal conditions, growing from an embryo to a mature adult that is ready to reproduce. However, when conditions turn harsh—such as a lack of food or extreme heat—the worm enters a state known as *dauer*. In this state, the worm's growth halts, its metabolism slows to nearly imperceptible levels, and it essentially "hibernates" until conditions improve. It can remain like this for years, waiting for the environment to signal that it's safe to resume its life cycle.

This concept of entering a survival state isn't unique to nematode worms. Many animals, including mammals, utilize hibernation or similar strategies to endure unfavorable conditions. For instance, bears gorge themselves in preparation for the winter months when food is scarce and they must conserve energy. Other creatures, like snails, protect themselves from extreme heat by closing up and entering a dormant state known as *estivation*. In essence, when survival is at risk, nature finds a way to pause, conserve and protect.

Now of course you're not the same as a worm or a bear, but there's a growing belief that chronic fatigue syndrome is a form of biological hibernation—your body's way of hitting "pause" to survive what it perceives as a dangerous environment.

We just need to appropriately indicate to your brain and body that they are safe. The baseline framework is one of the safest and most effective protocols to achieve this without making you feel worse.

THE BODY'S SURVIVAL MECHANISM

We humans have incredible brains. In fact, the human brain is divided into three parts: the executive center, the limbic system, and the reptilian brain.

The executive center is our most advanced part, responsible for creativity, critical thinking and reasoning.

The limbic system processes emotions and stress, acting as a bridge between our higher thoughts and our survival instincts.

The reptilian brain, the most primitive part, governs basic survival responses, including the fight-or-flight mechanism.

Here's the catch: your reptilian brain doesn't know the difference between life-threatening danger, like being chased by a predator, and everyday stress, such as losing your car keys or missing a deadline. It responds to all stress with the same biological cocktail of adrenaline, noradrenaline, and cortisol. While this fight-or-flight response can save your life in acute situations, chronic exposure to stress can overwhelm your body.

Dr. Lesslar brings in the work of Dr. Robert Naviaux, who developed the theory of the cell danger response (CDR). According to this theory, when the body is constantly bombarded with stress signals—whether from environmental factors, poor nutrition, or lack of sleep—it activates a protective response. In a state of constant danger, the body may enter a kind of biological hibernation, much like the nematode worm in *dauer*. This could explain the hallmark symptoms of CFS, such as fatigue, brain fog and exercise intolerance. The body, unable to distinguish between minor daily stresses and genuine threats, shuts down to conserve energy and protect itself from further harm.

So, how can we signal to our nervous system that the danger has passed and it's safe to resume normal function? The answers may lie in mimicking the cues that nature provides to animals when it's time to come out of hibernation. And yes, although you aren't a bear or worm, you do have a nervous system that works to protect you, and the good news is you can coax your body out of this hyper-protective state. Kinda amazing, right?

So, here's how it's done...

Create a safe environment

Just as animals wait for favorable conditions, your body needs to feel safe before it allows recovery. Reduce stress wherever possible—whether that means setting boundaries, practicing mindfulness, or simply allowing yourself time to rest without guilt. Surround yourself with positive, uplifting people and minimize exposure to negativity.

This isn't always easy to do. In fact, setting a boundary with a loved one or removing yourself from a negative situation can be easier said than done. Having a support network around you or people and professionals to help you with this is vital.

Regular restorative movement

Small, gentle movements can signal to your body that it's okay to come out of its dormant state. This doesn't mean jumping into an intense exercise routine, but it could be light movement that is appropriate based on where you're at. If you are in stage 1 of recovery, this could be sitting up in bed. Or doing some light movements from your bed, or simply moving to a different room during the day. We cover this much deeper in chapter 9, Movement; but for the later stages 1,2 and 3—short walks, stretching or restorative strength building movements done appropriately and within your capacity, helps a lot. Obviously the more you progress the more life opens up and you can do a lot more.

Sunlight and nature

Animals emerge from hibernation with the change in seasons, as warmer weather and longer daylight hours signal a shift in conditions. Exposure to natural sunlight helps regulate your circadian rhythm, boosting your energy levels and promoting better sleep.

Nourishing your body

Like a bear gorging on food before hibernation, your body needs consistent nourishment to feel secure. Eating a healthy, balanced nutrition plan can signal that you›re no longer in a state of famine or deprivation. A key tip here is to not wait to be hungry to eat. Eat regardless of hunger, especially initially. Meal frequency helps satiate the brain and body and regulate blood sugar levels so you feel calmer and more relaxed throughout the day.

Positive reinforcement

Your reptilian brain is in survival mode, but you can reassure it with positive thoughts and affirmations. By consciously focusing on safety and abundance, you may help retrain your brain and body to see the world as a less threatening place.

It's important to remember that recovery from CFS is not instantaneous. Just as a bear doesn't leap out of hibernation at the first sign of spring, your body may take time to adjust to the idea that it's safe to resume normal function. The key is to approach this process gently, with patience and kindness. Rushing or forcing yourself to "snap out of it" can backfire, reinforcing the body's need to protect itself.

By understanding the body's survival mechanisms, we gain insight into why chronic fatigue syndrome behaves the way it does. While the hibernation analogy may not be a perfect fit, it provides a useful framework for conceptualizing what's happening within your body.

Nature is always seeking balance, and in time and with the right support, your body can find its way out of its protective state and into recovery.

Nurturing that process, one small, supportive action at a time is key. Recovery is not about fighting against your symptoms; it's about creating a safe environment that allows your body to heal at its own pace.

And how do we do that?

1. Find your baseline!
2. Be consistent.
3. Enjoy your baseline.

WHAT ABOUT BASELINE SETBACKS?

Yes, there will be times when life gets in the way. As the common adage says, "Life is what happens while you're busy making other plans." There'll be circumstances that derail your best-laid plans. But the good news is—we have a full strategy for overcoming setbacks. You can read about it in chapter 10.

Whether you're feeling a dip in energy or you're experiencing a true setback, it's okay. Life isn't predictable and no one is immune to common setbacks. It's like a speed-hump in the road, it may give you a bump but it doesn't mean you stop driving towards your destination. Whether that's a cold or flu or a change in life circumstances, setbacks are a normal part of recovery, but with the right tools and support, you can bounce back sooner.

Enjoying Your Baseline

Your baseline is a place to enjoy. I often tell my clients to fall in love with their baseline. And they think I'm crazy. But if you can't fall in love with it, at least fall in like with it. Because the truth is, it's not always easy. Enjoying it or leaning into your current capacity and baseline takes courage, even when it feels impossible to do so. This doesn't happen overnight, but when I see clients take this advice on board, recovery starts to emerge. That means waking up each day with a sense of meaning, comfort, and appreciation for the small, steady rhythms of your life. It's tempting to chase only the end goal of "being recovered," but there is immense value in learning to love the simple, day-to-day moments.

Fall in love with the process

Famous NBA basketball player Lebron James once said in an interview, "The process is the only thing that matters to me. You know, I think when you fall in love with the process of what you want to do…The end result will happen organically, and it'll make it so much more worth your while when you fall in love with the process."

Now, we're not all mentally wired like sporting star—Lebron James, but we can share the same attitude towards our own goals. And **that is being process driven…and then, the outcome will come.**

Enjoying your baseline grounds you, reduces stress, and helps build emotional resilience. It allows you to feel more in control of your life and creates a foundation for long-term wellbeing. Now that's worth some inner celebration. Yes, celebrate your wins and the progress you make along the way. Feeling control is an empowering emotional state to be in when you have felt anything but that in the past.

Having a consistent routine and structure is crucial. Without it, you may feel directionless and reactive rather than intentional.

I like to ask my clients, "Do you run the day, or does the day run you?" When you don't have a plan or clear focus, the day can slip away in distractions, leaving you feeling unfulfilled. But by creating a baseline you enjoy—a healthy morning ritual, nourishing meals, time for rest and movement—you're more likely to feel fulfilled and happy with your progress journey. Ways to enjoy your baseline:

Start your day with gratitude: Write down three things you're thankful for every morning and one thing you're looking forward to doing that day to anchor your mindset.

Create a routine you genuinely like: Include simple things that bring you joy throughout the day, whether that be a morning ritual, being outside, listening to your favorite song, meditation or prayer, or looking over your vision board and goals to keep you focused.

Check in with yourself daily: Take a few moments to pause and ask, *How do I feel?* and *What do I need?* During hard times, I love the question: *What would self love do?*

Celebrate the little wins: Acknowledge small and big accomplishments, like making your bed or cooking a homemade meal. It's important to celebrate the wins. Every single Friday in our Mentorship recovery program we ask our members to do a check- in with us called "Friday wins." They share their wins for the week, or their lessons and insights. This helps with accountability and long-term progress.

Curate your environment: Make your space comfortable and inspiring. Whether that be rearranging your bedroom, throwing out old clothes or things that don't serve you anymore, decluttering, putting images or pictures of things that inspire you. Even paintings or plants can help too. Create a space that feels good for you.

Set daily intentions: Even just one focus or goal for the day can help you feel more in control. For example, a five minute meditation, or some time just being (no phone/no distractions) or if the laundry has been staring at you for three days (or more, we don't judge!), make it your goal to fold and put it away. Doing this one thing will give you a boost because you set the intention and then did it.

Practice presence: Try to notice the small pleasures of everyday life: the taste of your food, a moment of stillness, the feel of fresh air.

Enjoying your baseline doesn't mean settling—it means cultivating a life you like now (even if small initially) as you work toward where you want to be. It's the foundation for sustainable wellbeing.

MICHELLE

When I first met Michelle in 2014, she was in a world of pain. Physically, emotionally, cognitively and spiritually. In her own words, she was actually ready to give up. For the past decade, Michelle had been cooped up in her bedroom in Portland, Oregon. A beautiful beach town located on the west coast of the USA, yet she was too sick to even look out her bedroom window let alone go down to her local beach.

Michelle was in her 50s, she had some terrible life events happen to her, and then she had viruses/infections and literally two pages of other health conditions on top of chronic fatigue syndrome. She was so unwell that her mom, who was in her eighties, had to care for her.

Despite trying lots of different treatments and spending over $50,000 on things that didn't work, Michelle was severely ill when she came to CFS Health for help. She had tried everything from blood infusions and antivirals to other symptom management techniques. She was in a state of despair. She was very isolated, as her social life had come to a complete stop and her brain and body went into hibernation mode. Her skin was gray. Meals would get delivered to her bedroom by her mother. Michelle was well and truly in the red zone.

She had been in the vicious cycle of the first three recovery readiness zones from the giving up zone to the seeking zone. She'd spent thousands of dollars on stuff that didn't work. She was fed up with trying new things and she was ready to give up altogether.

On the first call we had together, she said to me, "There is nothing I can do." And so, the first thing we needed to do was create a baseline that was appropriate for her and within her capacity.

I said, "Michelle, you need to write a list of things you can do. No matter how small, what can you do at the moment?"

She responded that she could sit up out of bed for a few minutes at a time, go to the toilet once or twice a day and move her feet up and down while in bed. I got her to write a list of all the things that she could do on a daily basis and over time, the list grew.

Within a month, Michelle was sitting up in bed most of the time and she realized that she could put makeup on. Even though she wasn't going out, it brightened up her day and she kept doing it. She also started to make a structured routine based on what she could do, and in between doing things, she also allowed for rest.

Her sleep improved, her nutrition improved, her daily function improved. Therefore, her mood improved and her whole life started to improve. Her body naturally started to re-condition.

Within two months, I could see a difference in the color of her eyes and skin (a tangible sign of health coming back). She seemed a lot happier, and she started to look forward to the future. Within six months, Michelle had achieved some of the goals that she had set on her initial recovery plan call, including going downstairs to have her meals with her mother, wander around her garden and smell the roses, and go to the beach, put her feet in the water and enjoy the sand between her toes.

Within twelve months, she was walking twenty minutes along the beach most days. And within a year and a half, she was able to drive seven hours to see her best friend that she hadn't been able to see for ten years.

All this was possible because she focused on what she could do and didn't wait for recovery to happen. She started with where she was at. She stopped focusing on symptom-focused treatments that were keeping her stuck and instead she started doing the work and the work started paying off.

Again, consistency over intensity is the key to moving forwards.

Michelle is a perfect example of how even if you are at the point of giving up, it is possible to get into the green zone and eventually get your life back! Ten years on and she's still doing well. She's started her own business and has a whole new lease on life.

TAKEAWAYS

THE PUSH-CRASH CYCLE: Many people with CFS experience the push-crash cycle, where bursts of energy lead to overexertion and then a painful crash. The concept of a "baseline" was introduced, which is key to avoiding this cycle and making steady, sustainable progress by staying consistent with energy usage.

ESTABLISHING A BASELINE: Over two weeks, document key factors like sleep, meals, energy levels, and activities to create your baseline. Using this data, we will develop an "Imperfect, Perfect Daily Routine" that focuses on consistency, not perfection, and includes activities that energize you while avoiding energy drainers. The goal is to gradually build your capacity through small, consistent efforts without pushing beyond your current limits, allowing for steady progress toward recovery.

ENJOY YOUR BASELINE: Recovery is a journey, so make sure you find moments of joy throughout your recovery. This will keep you moving forward and help tremendously with your healing.

RECOVERY INSPIRATION

Download our free training to learn how to stop the Push-Crash Cycle, find your baseline and get back on track to recovery. In this training, you will figure out your baseline and how to start building consistency in your life!

CHAPTER 7

Get Mindset Ready

SET YOURSELF UP FOR SUCCESS

Mindset plays a powerful role in how we experience and respond to life—it shapes our outlook, our habits, and even our brain chemistry. But when it comes to chronic fatigue syndrome, it's important to be clear: this is *not* a matter of willpower or "toughing it out."

CFS is a complex neurological and immune condition, involving dysfunction in the body's energy systems, nervous system regulation, and immune response. It's a real, physiological illness—not a mindset problem.

That said, let's face it, going through chronic fatigue syndrome is freaking hard, extremely freaking hard. And it affects you mentally and emotionally.

Often people ask me what I do for work, and when I tell them that I help people with CFS get healthy and start living again, they often say, "Isn't that for people who are just depressed?" They comment as if it's a mindset problem.

And my response back to them is, "No CFS is a neurological illness that affects the brain and the body. It very much is a physical illness. However it does affect people physically and emotionally. Secondary anxiety and depression can occur for people with CFS because wouldn't you be pretty upset if tomorrow I took away all things you love and you couldn't do them any more, even though you wanted to?"

That always stops them in their tracks. They often reply with the same comment, "Oh that would be horrible, I'd hate that."

So while mindset can't *cure* CFS, it can influence how the brain and body cope.

Approaches that cultivate calm, acceptance, and self-compassion—rather than pushing or denying symptoms—can help reduce stress signals in the nervous system. This can make a massive difference in how your body functions day to day.

Cultivating a healthy mindset towards your recovery isn't about forcing positivity or pretending everything is fine. No one wants to hear another cheap, "just think positive," mantra. And we know there's no magical potion that will spontaneously heal CFS. But what we do know is that working *with* the brain and body and not against it plays an important role in our ability to recover.

Mindset shifts such as:

- Recognizing your capacity and limits without losing hope.
- Looking after yourself without guilt.
- Nurturing self-belief in your capacity to adapt.

- Believing that recovery is possible.
- Staying focused on your life now, not what it used to be.
- Letting go of negative beliefs that no longer serve you.
- Becoming aware and building presence into your day so you feel more peaceful.
- Not letting symptoms perpetuate into anxiety loops.
- Letting go of the old to build the new.

Mindset becomes less about "fighting" the illness, or staying caught in the trap of pushing and crashing, and more about creating conditions for healing, resilience, and personal growth. That way, you can become the new 2.0 version of yourself that is healthy and well.

ACCEPTANCE AND IDENTITY

At the beginning of this book I really dug into acceptance. I said "Acceptance is the first step to recovery." And it's true. Without accepting your situation and health condition, you can't move forward. Why?

Because you can't change what you refuse to acknowledge.

CFS feels unpredictable, limiting, and deeply frustrating. Many people can't accept their situation and push themselves to "soldier through". But this constant internal battle keeps you stuck in the cycle of denial of your reality and keeps you sick for longer. As I always say to my clients, if something is not working, change it. Keep doing what works but just important stop doing what doesn't work.

Acceptance means:

- Recognizing the illness is real.
- Acknowledging your current capacity.
- Letting go of the guilt around resting.
- Focusing on the present and what you can control.

Acceptance creates the environment for recovery. When you accept where you are, you have the ability to start your recovery journey.

Acceptance isn't the cure of course; it's what allows your healing to begin. Acceptance is what I call the bridge between being stuck and stepping towards progress. It's not giving up; it's the opposite. It's saying, *This is where I am right now—and this is what I can do to start moving forward.*

When you stop resisting reality, you release an incredible amount of energy.

Let's face it, fighting keeps you tense and drained. Acceptance opens the door for change.

Before acceptance you may have pushed past your limits repeatedly, be consumed by self-blame and guilt, chase after "quick fixes" and the next "instant cure." After acceptance life is different. You make informed choices based on your long-term health, move at a pace that supports healing, build routines that slowly expand your energy and capacity.

I once had a client who was just not seeing any results. He was super angry and frustrated. He jumped on a coaching call and said. "Toby, I'm still not getting better. I'm trying, but nothing is working."

I dived deeper into what was going on for him by asking more questions about his situation.

He said, "Well I have two or three good days, then I overdo it and end up back at square one."

I asked him if he had fully accepted where he was currently at.

"No, of course not," he replied. "I don't want to accept where I am at. I just want my old life back."

And in a moment everything clicked.

I said," You do realize that because you're not accepting your current reality, you keep pushing beyond your capacity, red-lining, and falling backwards. And it's been seven months of this same cycle and you are still not progressing. If you start with where you are—which means accepting your current situation—you will stop chasing your old life and start building your new life."

His eyes lit up. He realized then and there that not accepting his situation was the very thing keeping him stuck. He realized he had a choice. It was a powerful conversation and it changed the trajectory of his life.

Identity

I have spoken a lot about identity and how I was challenged to accept my situation. I was always looking back, trying to retrieve my old life, my previous status as a basketball player and regain former fitness levels. I was a self-identified sports person and didn't know myself without this identity.

Obviously your identity may be different; you may identify as a mom or dad, an artist, a coach, an athlete, a CEO, a runner, a hiker, a person who loves life and is full of vitality and positivity. You may be a "social butterfly" or someone who loves creativity and adventure. But having CFS reshapes your identity in ways you never expected. Maybe you were always known as someone who could push through anything, someone who had endless lists, endless goals, endless drive.

Suddenly you wake up and sometimes can't even lift your head off the pillow. You look at the person you used to be—the one who was always moving, always accomplishing, the one everyone knew you for—and you feel a sharp distance, like you're watching an earlier version of yourself from far. The contrast is painful. You feel grief, confusion, maybe even shame. You wonder, *Who am I without all that strength? Who am I if I can't keep up with the life I built? Who am I if I can't be the person that everyone knows me for?*

CFS forces you to confront these questions and your identity because the person you were and the person you are now seem poles apart. But you're still you—just living inside a body that now has very different needs.

Your identity was once tied to what you could do. You were the one who carried others, stayed late, pushed harder, went further. It was easy to build your worth around productivity and reliability, because the world rewards those things. When your abilities suddenly shrink, the story you've told yourself about who you are becomes shaky.

You don't need toxic positivity. You don't need to pretend CFS isn't life-changing. But there *is* a mindset that can help you survive this and even discover parts of yourself that were hidden before.

Here are a few small mindset shifts I encourage.

1. Be gentle with yourself.

You are not lazy. You are not weak. Your body is fighting an invisible battle every day. Treating yourself with compassion isn't optional—it's medicine.

2. Let your identity stretch and shift.

You are more than your former abilities. You still have creativity, humor, empathy, intelligence, and depth—none of which depend on physical stamina (although you will have that too when you recover).

3. Honor your limits rather than fighting them.

This illness punishes pushing. Partner with your body instead of resisting it. Tuning into your body and participating fully in your recovery is the smartest thing you can do.

4. Celebrate the small victories.

Sitting up. Making a meal. Answering one message. These moments count now. They matter. They are proof that you're still moving forward.

5. Find meaning in new ways.

Maybe you can't do what you used to, but you can still connect, observe, think, feel, create, love. Your worth doesn't disappear just because your pace changes.

6. The power of right now and yet.

Maybe there are many things that you can't do right now, but that doesn't mean you can't do them in the future. Instead of saying you can't do something. Say, "I can't do this *yet*." It carries less weight and shows you the possibilities of the future.

REBUILDING YOURSELF

When you go through CFS, you begin to realize that you haven't lost your identity. You're redefining it. You're discovering a quieter kind of strength—one that doesn't come from pushing harder, but from listening, adapting, and staying present through uncertainty. I view going through CFS as much of a spiritual journey as a physical one. You learn things that can't be taught through a textbook. It deepens you in ways that many never experience in their lifetime.

You are not the same person you were before the illness. But you're not less.

You're becoming someone who knows resilience on a deeper level—someone whose value isn't earned through motion, but through existence. You are still here. You are still you. And that is enough. You are enough. You are worthy as you are.

New Life vs. Old Life

When you get sick, you don't just lose energy—you lose parts of yourself. You lose the version of you who could wake up and do things without thinking twice. It feels like one day, you had a life—and the next, it disappeared.

People often talk about physical symptoms, but few talk about the emotional pain of watching your old life fade away while you're still here. That kind of grief is deep. It's quiet. It's hard for others to see—but it's real.

It's okay to grieve. In fact, it's essential. Grief is not a sign of weakness; it's a sign of love. You're grieving the life, the people, and the version of yourself that meant something to you.

But some people get stuck in recovery because they're still trying to get back to their *old life*. They measure progress by how close they feel to their past self—the one who was productive, busy, and always achieving. But that version of you lived by different rules—rules that might have led you to CFS in the first place.

When you stop fighting and wasting energy on trying to get your old life back, you make space to build a new one. One that is more enriching and health producing.

~~~~~~

**You can't heal in the same
environment you got sick in.
You can only heal by becoming who you're
meant to be now, not who you were.**

~~~~~~

I remember the moment it happened for me. After years of trying to "get my old life back," I realized that I didn't actually want it. I didn't want to live in that same high-pressure, fast-paced, disconnected way. I wanted peace. I wanted balance. I wanted health, I wanted to wake up calm—not stressed, not chasing, not proving.

Building the New Life

Your new life starts small—one moment at a time. It begins when you stop asking, "When will I get my old life back?" and start asking, "What kind of life do I want to build?" This is your chance to create a life that's more aligned with who you really are—one that honors your health, your energy, your values, and your peace.

Ask yourself:

- *What matters to me most right now?*
- *Why is that important?*
- *Who do I want to be?*
- *Who do I want to become?*
- *What kind of people do I want around me?*

- *What kind of work, creativity, or contribution feels meaningful now?*
- *What does success mean to me today—not ten years ago?*
- *What does health look like for me now?*

You're not starting from zero. You're starting from wisdom and experience. From a deeper knowing of what truly matters. When you let go of your old identity—the achiever, the fixer, the helper, the perfectionist—it can feel like you're losing everything. But in truth, you're coming home to yourself.

You start redefining who you are beyond what you *do*. You begin to realize you are not your productivity, your energy level, or your illness. You are the awareness behind it all—the one choosing, learning, and growing through it.

That realization changes everything. It's where real freedom begins.

You must let go of the old to build the new.

Letting Go and Trusting the Unknown

Letting go is uncomfortable. It feels like stepping into an empty space—a gap between who you were and who you're becoming. That in-between is sacred. It's where the new life is born. But it does require courage, which I will touch on deeper at the end of this book.

EXERCISE

Grab a pen and draw two columns in your journal.

In the first column, write **"My Old Life."** List what defined you back then—your routines, beliefs, values, habits, and expectations.

In the second column, write **"My New Life."** Now list what you want to carry forward— and what you're ready to leave behind.

Here's an example to get you started:

My Old Life	My New Life
Overdoing, ignoring my body	Listening, responding with care
Pleasing everyone	Setting gentle boundaries
Living for others' approval	Living from my own truth
Constant rush	Slower, intentional pace
Stress as normal	Calm as the baseline

As you do this, you'll notice that not everything from your old life needs to go. Some things—like kindness, passion, or creativity—will come with you. They just evolve into a healthier form.

You don't need to know every detail of what's next. You just need to keep taking gentle steps toward what is helpful right now.

It's easy to trip yourself up when you are looking at the mountain top. It can feel too hard, too big and too scary. But the truth is, you just need to look at the next step in front of you. Each step you take will get you closer to that beautiful mountain top. Eventually, over time you will get there if you do the right things at the right time, one step at a time.

THE POWER OF BELIEFS

Every belief you hold is a lens through which you experience life. It colors how you interpret your symptoms, your progress, and even your identity. When you've been unwell for a long time, your brain starts collecting evidence that supports the idea that you're broken. It remembers every crash, every setback, every time you couldn't keep up—and soon those memories harden into "truths."

- I'll never get better.
- My body is too fragile.
- No one understands me.
- I'm a burden.
- I'm too old.
- I'm not worthy.
- I'm different.

The problem isn't that you have these thoughts. It's that your mind begins to believe them. And the body responds to what the mind believes.

Every thought sends a chemical message through the body. When you think something fearful or hopeless, the body releases stress hormones—adrenaline, cortisol, noradrenaline—preparing you to fight, flee, or freeze. Over time, this keeps the nervous system in survival mode, preventing healing. But when you think a hopeful, safe, or encouraging thought, your brain releases a different cocktail—dopamine, serotonin, oxytocin—creating calm and connection.

Your beliefs literally shift your physiology.

The groundbreaking work of cell biologist Dr. Bruce Lipton shows that our biology is shaped by our beliefs.[5] That we aren't just hardwired by genetics but in fact, our environment, our thoughts, and the way we perceive life can influence the way our bodies react and develop. The body doesn't know whether a thought is "true"—it simply responds as if it is. This is why shifting belief isn't wishful thinking; it's rewiring your biology. Therefore, I believe it's important to examine our beliefs and assess which ones are useful to keep and which ones are useful to let go of. Here are a few I hear often.

"I'm different."
I hear this all the time when people think they are the exception to recovering. You might experience different symptoms, but that

doesn't make recovery impossible. I've seen people with complex cases get better. Ask yourself—*is this belief enhancing or hindering me?*

"I need to find the problem."

Testing and data are useful to rule out major issues—but once you've done that, endlessly searching for "the root problem" keeps you stuck. Put that energy back into building yourself up, to focusing on what you can do to get better, rather than getting stuck down rabbit holes with no solutions.

"I need to fix my symptoms."

Here's something powerful: when I asked a group of 150 clients whether focusing on symptoms ever helped, not one raised their hand. When I asked who felt better when focusing on *enhancing health*, every hand went up. **Enhancing is always better than obsessing over symptoms.** Ask yourself: *Is this enhancing me or hindering me?*

Backwards vs. Forwards Thinking

When we examine our beliefs and thinking. I often ask my clients to become aware of the state of mind they spend their time in. Is it backwards or forwards thinking?

Backwards thinking sounds like:

- Will this work for me?
- I'm different.
- I need to find the problem.
- I need to fix my symptoms.

That's fear-based, reactive, and it keeps you stuck.

Forwards thinking sounds like:

- What can I do to help myself today?
- What can I learn from this?
- How can I move closer to what I want?

And here's the key:

It's not just the *thought*—it's the *behavior* that follows it. If you think, *This won't work for me,* then you won't act. If you think, *What's my next best step?*—you'll take one. On a bigger scale, if you believe that recovery is not possible, you will resign to thinking there is nothing you can do and lose power over the situation. On the other hand, if you believe recovery is possible for you, you will start to do things that enhance your health and in return, feel more empowered.

Thoughts create behavior, and behavior creates results.

The Brain and Belief

The brain learns through repetition and emotion. Every time you think a thought with strong feeling behind it, neurons wire together—"what fires together, wires together."

If you've repeated "I'm stuck," hundreds of times, your brain has built a strong neural highway that supports that belief. But the beauty of neuroplasticity is that you can build a new one at any time. The more you practice a new thought—even if you don't fully believe it yet—the stronger that new pathway becomes. Eventually, it becomes the automatic default.

That's why this work takes daily awareness. You're not trying to erase old beliefs overnight; you're teaching your brain a new language of possibility. Every day, we run an internal dialogue—quiet, automatic, and powerful. It's that stream of thoughts asking questions like, *What's wrong with me?* or *Why can't I just feel normal?*

Most people never stop to notice these questions. Yet, they shape the direction of our mind, our focus, and ultimately, how we feel.

When things go wrong, we tend to ask really bad questions. We spiral into *Why me?*, *What's wrong with me?*, or *Why can't I fix this?* And our brain, doing its job, begins to search for answers to those questions—often finding only more fear, guilt, or self-blame. This creates a feedback loop that reinforces suffering. The quality of your life will always reflect the quality of the questions you ask yourself.

Analyzing Your Current Questions

Start by observing your current internal dialogue.

Grab a pen and paper and write down the things you ask yourself each day. Don't filter or judge. This simple act gets the clutter out of your head and onto paper where you can finally see it clearly. You might notice questions like: *What's wrong with me? Why do I feel this way? Why can't I be normal again?*

Once you've written them down, read them out loud. You'll quickly see how harsh, repetitive, or unhelpful they are. We do this to create distance—so we can look at our thinking instead of being lost inside it.

Shifting Focus: Negative vs. Empowering Questions

When you catch yourself asking questions that lead you deeper into despair, pause and replace them with better ones.

Here's how to shift your focus:

Negative Question	Empowering Question
"What's wrong with me?"	"What can I do right now that would help me feel a little better?"
"Why is this happening to me?"	"What is this teaching me?"
"Why does no one understand?"	"How can I show myself the understanding I need?"
"Why is this so hard?"	"What's the message in the mess?"
"When will this end?"	"What small progress can I make today?"

Every time you redirect a question, you re-train your mind to look for solutions instead of problems.

Your brain is like a search engine it finds whatever you ask it to find. Ask negative questions, and it will collect evidence to prove that you're broken. Ask constructive questions, and it will find evidence that healing and progress are possible.

You Must Stay Curious

A curious mindset will allow you to be open to different possibilities, a conclusive mindset however will keep you closed off to anything other than the current reality you are experiencing.

I always say that our current reality is a reflection of our current thoughts, behaviors, actions or inactions. And so we must identify what's working and what's not working. What we need to do more of and what we need to do less of. This is why a curious mindset is so important.

I once had a client called Mary. When she jumped on her initial enrollment call to join the online recovery program, she was super excited. She knew she needed to work on her baseline to stop the ups and downs, she knew she needed help with her nutrition and restorative movement, and she was ready for it.

Until the moment she was about to sign and pay for the program.

She said, "Toby, I don't think I can do this."

I said, "What do you mean Mary? We just spent the last 50 minutes going over your health assessment and everything I said that you need to work on, you agreed with. What has changed?"

"Toby, I need my husband to understand me and my illness before I get better. He needs to understand my situation in order for me to get better."

I said, "My god Mary, if that's the case, you might be waiting for a very long time. If you need to wait for another human being to understand your condition for you to get better, what if he never fully understands it? Are you still going to wait?

"Ahhh you got me Toby, you're right to sign me up." Mary said.

I said, "No Mary, this isn't about me getting you. This is about you deciding to put yourself first, this is about you not waiting for someone else's approval or full understanding for you to do something about it. It's your choice, but if you think you need your husband to fully understand your condition (which he won't because he has never experienced CFS) you're going to remain stuck. What if it was possible to get better, regardless if your husband understands CFS or not?"

Mary joined the program that day, and because she had a curious mindset she was able to set herself free from the constraints of thinking that had kept her stuck for a very long time.

I'm happy to share that Mary did recover, and her husband was pleased to have his wife healthy and well again.

Creating New Beliefs and Action Plans

Once you've identified limiting beliefs, you can't just leave a blank space—you need to consciously build new ones.

Start by asking:

- *What do I want to believe instead?*
- *What thoughts would serve my highest values and future self?*
- *How can I live these beliefs through daily actions?*

Your Tongue Holds Power

Speaking more of what you want into your world will not only change how you feel physiologically, but also help you move towards your goals faster.

Have you ever noticed people who complain a lot about their lives and circumstances are always the same, nothing ever changes. They are constantly focusing on what they don't want, focusing on what they don't like, and yet they continue to have more of what they don't want.

You can do the opposite, use your words wisely, share verbally more of what you want, state how you do want to feel, speak life to more of what you want. Where focus goes, energy flows.

Linking your words with the possibility of what you want more (combined with action) will help you create the reality you want. As the great quote by philosopher Ludwig Wittgenstein says "The limits of my language mean the limits of my world."

EXERCISE
THE NEW BELIEF BUILDER

1. Write down an old belief that's not serving you.
   Example: "I'll never get better."

2. Replace it with a new belief.
   Example: "My body is capable of healing."

3. Write **three actions** that align with your new belief.
   Example:
   - I will rest before I crash.
   - I will nourish my body with care.
   - I will acknowledge small progress daily.

Every time you act in alignment with a new belief, you prove it to yourself. Belief becomes behavior. Behavior becomes habit. Habit becomes reality.

Remember: change doesn't come from thinking about it—it comes from living it, one small step at a time.

GUILT

Guilt is one of the heaviest emotions people carry during chronic illness. It's not just emotional—it's physical. It sits in your chest, in your gut, in your muscles. It makes you feel tight, stuck, and drained.

You might feel guilty for not being who you used to be.

Guilty for not doing enough.

Guilty for saying no.

Guilty for needing help.

I remember when I was going through CFS, I felt deeply guilty for being sick. My family and I were trying everything to get better and every time something didn't work, I felt horrible. It felt like I was letting them down. Every day I would wake up feeling guilty that "I wasn't better yet."

Guilt can become so normal that you don't even notice it's there anymore—like a low hum in the background. But it quietly eats away at your peace, your progress, and your confidence.

Today, we start unpacking that weight.

Understanding Guilt

Guilt isn't all bad. It's a signal—a sign that something matters to you. It tells you when you've acted out of alignment with your values. That kind of guilt can guide you back to integrity. But the kind of guilt most people with chronic illness experience isn't helpful. It's *false guilt*—guilt that comes from unrealistic expectations, fear of judgment, and pressure to please everyone.

This kind of guilt doesn't come from your values—it comes from other people's. Let's look at how this plays out.

You have a belief: *I should be doing more.* That belief triggers behavior—maybe you push yourself even when your body is screaming for rest. Then, when you crash, you feel guilty for not being able to keep up. So, to silence that guilt, you push again.

And the cycle repeats.

Belief → Behavior → Burnout → Guilt → Belief (again)

That's the External Guilt Loop. It's powered by the fear of disappointing others, the need for approval, or the old identity of being "the capable one."

Breaking free starts when you question the belief that created it.

Layers of Guilt

There are many layers to guilt. Some are surface-level—the day-to-day "I should've done more" kind. Others run deeper—tied to identity, worth, and belonging.

Let's explore the main layers:

1. **Guilt of Doing**—Feeling bad for resting, slowing down, or not being productive.
2. **Guilt of Being**—Feeling like a burden, ashamed for needing help, or not being your "old self."
3. **Inherited Guilt**—Taking on responsibility for others' emotions or expectations.
4. **Survivor's Guilt**—Feeling bad for improving when others are still suffering.

EXERCISE
BREAKING THE LOOP

Grab your journal and answer these questions honestly:

1. What are the things I feel most guilty about right now?
    Example: Resting, saying no, not earning money,
    missing social events?

2. Who taught me to feel guilty about those things?
    (Was it family, culture, society, or past
    experiences?)

3. What would it feel like to release that guilt—even
    for one day?
    (Freedom? Relief? Self-trust?)

4. What's one small action I can take that aligns with
    my truth, not my guilt?

5. What will my future self thank me for?

The Backpack of Expectations

Imagine you're carrying a heavy backpack. Inside it are all the expectations—from family, friends, work, culture, society, and even yourself. You've been carrying it for so long that you forgot what it's like to feel freely.

Each expectation adds more weight:

- I should be better by now.
- I shouldn't need rest.
- I should be productive every day.
- I should always be there for others.

Now, close your eyes for a moment and imagine taking the backpack off.

Place it on the ground. Breathe. You don't have to carry it anymore. You can choose what stays in there and what goes.

What's most important is asking yourself: *Is holding on to any of this helpful?* If it is, keep it, if it's not you can lay it to rest and be at peace with yourself.

EXERCISE
EMPTYING THE BACKPACK

- Write down all the "shoulds" and expectations you're carrying.
  Example: *I should be more social. I should look healthier. I should have it figured out. I should be better by now. I should be fitter.*

- Circle the ones that don't belong to you—the ones you inherited from others.

- Cross them out. Say out loud: "This doesn't belong to me anymore. This isn't mine to carry, this doesn't serve me anymore."

- Rewrite the remaining ones as **truths** that empower you. Example:
  - "I should rest." → "I'm allowed to rest."
  - "I should be productive." → "Resting is productive."
  - "I should be better." → "I'm improving in my own time."

This is how you begin to
redefine success on your own terms.

The Guilt and Worth Connection

Guilt often hides a deeper story—one about worth. If you grew up believing love had to be earned, then rest, ease, and self-care might feel "wrong."

But your worth is not up for debate. You are valuable because you exist—not because of what you do or how much you give.

Healing happens when you start treating yourself with the same compassion you give to everyone else. Let's take this deeper. When you remove guilt, what remains is truth—the quiet voice underneath all the noise.

Ask yourself:

- *What do I actually want and need right now?*
- *What do I believe is right for me?*
- *What kind of life do I want to create moving forward?*

You'll notice that your truth is never harsh or demanding. It's calm. It's gentle. It's kind. It doesn't guilt you into change—it invites you into it.

Read these slowly, aloud if you can:

- I am not responsible for everyone else's feelings.
- Rest is not weakness; it's wisdom.
- Saying no is a form of self-respect.
- I am allowed to receive care, love, and help.
- I do not need to earn my worth.
- I can be healing and still be enough.

Repeat them daily until they start to feel true.

The opposite of guilt isn't carelessness—it's self-respect. When you release guilt, you don't stop caring; you start caring from a place of truth instead of fear.

So the next time guilt whispers, *You're not doing enough,* smile softly and say, *I'm doing exactly what I need to heal.*

A brilliant question to help you get centered is. *What would self love do?* The answer will always bring you back on track.

PEOPLE-PLEASING

If you've spent most of your life putting others first, struggling to say no, or feeling guilty for taking care of yourself, this section is for you.

Pleasing-people is not kindness, it's fear wearing a smile. It's the habit of prioritizing everyone else's needs above your own in the hope that it will bring peace, approval, or love. But the truth is, people-pleasing drains your energy, weakens your boundaries, and keeps your nervous system in constant overdrive.

You can't heal when your energy is being spent trying to make everyone else comfortable.

How People-Pleasing Impacts Health

People-pleasing has deep physiological effects. It keeps your body in a state of *hypervigilance*—always scanning for how others are feeling, worrying about what they think, and adjusting your behavior to avoid conflict or disappointment. It's exhausting.

When your nervous system is constantly trying to manage everyone else's emotions, it has no energy left to restore your own. We try to fill up our cup of worth from outside of ourselves—and that cup never stays full.

This external validation loop means that every moment of peace depends on someone else's reaction. When people approve, you feel safe. When they don't, you crumble. And that instability keeps your body locked in stress mode. It's stressful even thinking about it.

Common Signs of People-Pleasing

If you're unsure whether this pattern applies to you, here are some signs from our workshops and client experiences:

- Constantly feeling anxious, unsettled, or guilty when you rest.
- Needing reassurance to make decisions.
- Fear of being disliked or misunderstood.
- Saying yes when you want to say no.
- Difficulty asking for or receiving help.
- Feeling resentful when your effort isn't appreciated.
- Feeling lost when you're not "needed" by others.

The root emotion behind all of this is **fear**—fear of rejection, fear of conflict, fear of not being enough.

The Hidden Need Behind People Pleasing

One of the most overlooked steps in overcoming people-pleasing is understanding what needs are being met. Every behavior—even the unhelpful ones—is trying to meet a need. People-pleasing often meet needs for love, connection, safety, or significance. On some level, it's your nervous system's way of saying, *If I can make everyone happy, I'll stay safe.*

It's not wrong. It's just outdated. This strategy might have protected you once—in childhood, in relationships, in environments where love had to be earned.

But as an adult, it becomes a cage. When you learn to meet those needs from within through self-compassion, boundaries, and truth—you stop needing external approval to feel whole.

The Cost of Control

People pleasers often feel a sense of *control* by managing how others see them.

If I act a certain way, they'll think I'm kind, capable, or worthy.

But this control is an illusion. It keeps you trapped in constant anxiety—walking on eggshells, afraid that if you stop pleasing, you'll lose love. And when others don't reciprocate your energy, you feel resentful. Not because you're unkind but because you've been giving from emptiness.

Resentment—The Silent Alarm

A key sign that you're over-pleasing is resentment. It's the body's way of saying, *I've given too much.* When your giving isn't reciprocated, or when you keep saying yes out of obligation, resentment builds. It's not anger at others—it's anger at yourself for abandoning your own needs.

EXERCISE
AWARENESS AND OWNERSHIP

Take a moment to journal through these prompts:

1. What am I afraid will happen if I stop pleasing everyone?

2. Who taught me that saying no was selfish or wrong?

3. In what moments do I ignore my needs to make others comfortable?

4. What am I trying to gain through people-pleasing—love, peace, control, approval?

5. How else could I meet that need in a healthier way?

Write freely. Awareness is the first act of self-liberation.

Resentment is not a flaw; it's feedback. It shows you where boundaries are missing.

Boundaries Begin With You

Boundaries are not about controlling others—they're about protecting your peace. Most people communicate boundaries through what they *don't want*:

"Stop doing that."

"You always make me feel..."

But this approach keeps everyone guessing. True boundaries come from clarity, not criticism. You can't set a boundary until you know what you want. Ask yourself: *What is actually important to me that's not being honored right now? Is it respect? Patience? Communication? Rest?"*

Once you know your need, communicate it clearly and calmly.

**Boundaries don't work when you
only express what's wrong.
They work when you express what's right for you.**

For example, instead of saying, "You never give me space," try, "I need some quiet time to rest after work. I'll message you later tonight."

This way, you're empowering both yourself and the other person. You're teaching them how to respect you—not through guilt, but through honesty.

Boundaries are an act of love—for you and for others.

From Pleasing to Peaceful

At first, setting boundaries feels uncomfortable. Your mind will panic: *They'll be upset!* Your body might shake. You'll second-guess. That's normal. It's your nervous system learning safety in truth.

Start small:

- Say no to one small thing this week.
- Take ten minutes of rest even if the house isn't perfect.
- Allow someone else to help you.

Each time you choose truth over guilt, you rewire your brain for peace.

You don't need to stop caring about others—you just need to care for yourself *too*. Parents often ask me, "Toby, how can I put myself first when I have kids to look after?"

I reply, "If you can't put yourself first, at least put yourself equal." That's fair.

True kindness comes from fullness, not emptiness. When you please everyone but yourself, you lose connection with who you really are. When you start honoring your needs, your relationships become more real—based on truth, not performance. You don't have to betray yourself to be loved.

The right people will love the real you.

THE PERFECTIONIST TRAP

Many CFS sufferers are self-proclaimed perfectionists. Trying extra hard. Wanting to do it all perfectly—diet, supplements, health, every task.

The stress of perfectionism is often worse than the thing you're trying to fix.

Being a perfectionist may have been one of your strengths. You held yourself to high standards, worked hard, showed up fully, and took pride in doing things *right*. You liked being the person who others could count on—the one who went the extra mile, who didn't settle for "good enough," who finished what they started.

Now, suddenly perfectionism feels like a heavy weight you could barely drag behind you. Maybe now even the simplest tasks sometimes take more energy than you have. Something that used to take you twenty minutes might take hours, or days, or simply never get done. You make plans you can't follow through on. You start things you can't finish. You lose track of commitments. And each time it happens, that old perfectionist voice tries to shame you:

Why can't you do more? Why can't you push harder? Why can't you be who you were before? It's not good enough!

Perfectionism and CFS clash in the hardest way—because perfectionism demands control, consistency, and performance… and CFS takes all three. Living with both feels like a tug-of-war inside your mind:

- You want to do everything well, and at 100%, but your body wants to rest.
- You want to meet expectations, but your energy sometimes doesn't allow it.
- You want to keep your standards high, but your reality forces them lower.

Being a perfectionist isn't your enemy—it means you care deeply. It means you have pride, discipline, passion. The problem is when you *punish yourself* about it.

Your standards don't have to disappear but they do need to adapt to your current reality. Sometimes "good enough" is actually heroic. Sometimes resting is the most disciplined choice you can make.

Recovering from CFS forces you to rewrite the rules you've lived by, and that's incredibly hard for a perfectionist heart. But you don't need to do everything right now. **Pick what you need now and move forwards.**

Progress over perfection. Stop the torturous self-pressure and expectation.

Be kind to yourself.

Again, ask, *what would self love do?*

BOUNDARIES

Boundaries are one of the most powerful tools for emotional, physical, and mental healing. Without boundaries, you feel scattered, resentful, and exhausted. You overextend, overgive, and override your own needs to avoid conflict. With boundaries, you begin to feel calm, grounded, and safe in your own energy again.

Most people think boundaries are about keeping others out—they're not. They're about keeping yourself *intact*.

The Link Between Boundaries and Health

When you have weak or unclear boundaries, your nervous system never gets to rest.

You're constantly managing other people's emotions, trying to predict reactions, or bending to keep the peace. That keeps you stuck in a low-grade state of stress and alertness—which, over time, becomes fatigue, burnout, or illness.

Healthy boundaries regulate your nervous system. They signal safety to your body by saying: *I can protect my energy. I can choose what I allow in. I'm safe to rest.*

In recovery, this isn't optional—it's essential.

The Three Elements of Boundaries

Every healthy boundary has three key parts:

1. Setting the Boundary—Defining Your Need
2. Communicating the Boundary—Expressing It Clearly
3. Honoring the Boundary—Following Through Consistently

Let's break these down

1. Setting Boundaries—Defining Your Need

You can't set a boundary until you know what you want. This might sound simple, but many people don't know what they actually need—they only know what they *don't* want.

You might say:

"I don't want people to take advantage of me."

"I don't want to feel drained all the time."

"I don't want to be left out."

But that's not a boundary—it's a complaint. Boundaries come from clarity. Instead of focusing on what you don't want, ask: *What do I want instead?*

- I want to be treated with respect. This is what respect looks like for me...
- I want time to recharge before social events. I will need one hour on my own to calm and regulate my nervous system.
- I want to communicate honestly without fear. Before you share how you feel, can you listen to what I have to share?

2. Communicating the Boundary—Saying It Out Loud

You can't expect people to honor needs you haven't expressed. No one is a mind reader.

Communicating a boundary doesn't have to be harsh or defensive—it can be kind, clear, and calm. When you express what you *do* want rather than what you *don't*, people are more likely to understand and respect it.

Here's how to shift your language:

Instead of saying...	Try saying...
"You never give me space."	"I need some quiet time after work. I'll message you later tonight."
"You always dump things on me."	"I can't take that on right now, but I hope you find the support you need."
"Stop asking me for help all the time."	"I love supporting you, but I need a break today to rest and recharge."

You don't have to explain, justify, or over-apologize. Your boundaries are valid because they protect your wellbeing.

3. Honoring Boundaries—The Follow-through

Setting and communicating boundaries is one thing. Honoring them is where the real growth happens. When you break your own boundaries, you teach people that your words aren't real. When you honor them, you build *self-trust*.

Honoring means you don't abandon yourself, even when it's uncomfortable. You stay consistent, calm, and compassionate—even if others don't like it.

Remember you are not responsible for other people's reactions. Their disappointment doesn't mean you did something wrong. Saying "no" to them is saying "yes" to your health.

At first, it might feel awkward or even scary—but with practice, it becomes strength.

Boundaries and Relationships

Healthy relationships are built on mutual respect—not sacrifice. When you start honoring your own limits, you'll quickly see who respects them and who resists them.

Some people will adjust beautifully. Others might push back. That doesn't mean your boundary is wrong—it means you're changing the pattern.

Stay gentle, but firm. Remember that your healing might make others uncomfortable—not because you're doing something bad, but because you're doing something *different*.

EXERCISE
THE BOUNDARY AUDIT

1. **Write down the areas of your life** where you feel resentful, drained, or taken advantage of.
   (Work, family, friendships, relationships, social media, etc.)

2. **Identify the common thread.**
   What value is being violated? (Respect, rest, honesty, time, space, fairness?)

3. **Write one sentence that defines your boundary** in that area.
   Example:
   - I need time alone after calls to rest.
   - I don't discuss my health with people who invalidate me.
   - I won't apologize for taking care of myself.

4. **Choose one boundary to practice this week.**
   Start small. Small wins build confidence.

Boundaries are not about control. They're about self-respect. Stating boundaries brings empowerment.

Boundaries can look like saying:
- "I'm not available for what hurts me anymore."
- "I am allowed to protect my peace."
- "You matter to me, and I matter to me, too."

And when you live from that place, your relationships actually become healthier because they're built on truth instead of guilt or obligation. Setting boundaries is one of the most courageous acts of healing. It requires honesty, self-awareness, and practice. You'll wobble at first—everyone does. But each time you uphold a boundary, you send a message to your nervous system that says, *I'm safe. I've got me.*

And that's where real peace begins.

There are boundaries for others and there are boundaries for yourself. I often get my clients to write out a list of both so they can stay consistent and focused on reaching their goals and dreams.

Boundaries for others are what we just went through above, boundaries for self, are about you—the habits and behaviors you want to do more of (or less of) for the benefit of your wellbeing.

Things like:

- I stick to regular sleep and wake times to feel more restored.
- I stay off social media between the hours of 6 a.m. and 6 p.m. so I create more time for peace and presence.
- I stay focused on my restorative movement and breathing exercises that make me feel good
- I eat healthy whole foods every three to four hours to fuel my body and brain.
- I say no to things that no longer serve me.

All these examples are boundaries for self and create discipline in a healthy way that will create more freedom long-term.

My old mentor Craig Harper used to ask "What are your non-negotiables?"

What he meant was, what are you committed to doing consistently that will ensure your success, despite the hardship and challenges that come your way. Regardless of whether motivation is there or not. What are your non-negotiables?

> **EXERCISE**
>
> Take a piece of paper now and write down a
> list of empowering boundaries for yourself
> that feel good for you.

YOUR VISION AND CREATING YOUR FUTURE

When you've been unwell for a long time, it's easy to lose sight of who you are beyond the illness. You stop dreaming. You stop planning. You start surviving. Creating your future vision is all about remembering that you still have a future.

> **"We run out of energy when
> we run out of vision."**
> **—Robin Sharma**

A vision isn't a fantasy or a wish list. It's a heartfelt picture of what life could look like if you lived from your truth—not fear, illness, or expectation.

Gemma said it beautifully in one of our workshops:

"When I made my first vision board, I was housebound. A good day meant sitting up for half an hour. But even then, I could dream. I could feel the joy of possibility—and that kept me going."

Your vision doesn't have to be big or flashy. It just needs to feel like *you and be more of what you'd like, in the future.*

This next process isn't about *goal setting* or ticking boxes. It's about rediscovering what matters to you and creating a life that aligns with your values, energy, and truth NOW.

Before we begin, let's get clear on what this process will help you do:

1. **Define your future** not in perfect detail, but with clarity and feeling. What would you like to be doing? How would you like to be feeling? (Remember to focus on what you want here, not what you don't want.)

2. **Learn how to visualize it**—so it feels real and inspiring. You can lay down and place your hands on your belly, close your eyes and allow your mind to visualize how it would feel to be living and doing the things you wrote down. Are you in nature? Surrounded by friends and family? What sounds can you hear? What smells can you smell? How does it feel in your body to be experiencing these things? You can smile while you are doing this visualization. A certain word might come to you, like peace, freedom, or calm. Enjoy it.

3. **Break it into timelines**—so you know what belongs to *now*, what's *next*, and what's *later*. This is where we reverse-engineer what you want to be doing into smaller bite-sizes pathways so you can get to your dreams. If one of your visions involves physical strength, then we need to create a restorative strength program for where you are at and build from there. If your vision involves having more cognitive capacity to socialize or use your brain power then we need to create a progressive plan for where you are at and build that up, so you can eventually do the thing you want to do.

Common pitfalls

Before creating your vision, here are some common pitfalls people make and how to avoid them.

1. **Overcomplicating it.**
2. Don't overthink or analyze every detail.
3. When you get stuck, ask yourself: *What's my best guess?*
4. This process is meant to be *fun*, not perfect.
5. **Putting too much pressure on yourself.**
6. You don't need to have all the answers today.
7. Life unfolds gradually—your vision will too.
8. **Being too serious.**
9. This is not a test or a report card.
10. Approach it with curiosity and playfulness.
11. **Trying to get it right.**
12. Your vision will evolve as you do.

13. What matters is how it feels—not how it looks.

14. **Focusing only on goals.**

15. This isn't about timelines or achievements.

16. It's about the feeling you want to wake up to each day.

The Six Key Areas of Life

When creating your vision, explore it across six key areas.
These represent a whole, balanced life—one built on meaning,
not just milestones.

1. Relationships

Think about the people who fill your life. Who supports and
uplifts you?

What kind of relationships do you want to nurture moving
forward—friendships, family, community, love?

Ask yourself:

- *What kind of energy do I want around me?*
- *How do I want to show up in my relationships?*
- *Who feels safe, supportive, and aligned with my growth?*

Healthy relationships are reciprocal. They don't drain; they restore.

2. Health

This isn't just about the absence of symptoms—it's about vitality.

Ask yourself:

- *What does health mean to me now?*
- *How does it feel in my body when I'm balanced?*
- *What habits help me feel grounded and alive?*

Health might look like daily rest, nourishing food, slow movement, laughter, sunlight, or time in nature. Whatever it is, define it on your own terms—not by society's standards.

3. Career, Business, and Contribution

Contribution is about purpose using your strengths and story to make a difference. It's not about working long hours or chasing success; it's about meaningful engagement with life.

Ask yourself:

- *What kind of work or endeavor would feel purposeful and energizing for me?*
- *How do I want to contribute to the world—even in small ways?*
- *What gifts or insights do I already have that could help others?*

You don't need to have the "big picture" now—just start with curiosity.

4. Personal Purpose

This is your why. The reason you get up in the morning—beyond obligations and expectations.

Your purpose doesn't have to be grand. It might be as simple as:

- To live peacefully.
- To inspire others by being real.
- To find joy in the little things.

Purpose gives direction when motivation fades.

5. Money and Wealth

Money is energy. It's a resource to help yourself and help others.

It supports your health, your lifestyle, freedom, and impact.

Ask yourself:

- *What does financial stability look like for me?*
- *What beliefs about money need to shift?*
- *How can I create security without stress?*

Money can enhance your life and the people around you that matter to you the most. It might be that money supports your health, with high quality food, a comforting place to live and an environment that helps you thrive over time. It also supports your dreams in arts, crafts, hobbies, business impact goals, or charities and passions that matter to you. It's about using it to improve your livelihood and well-being along with others you care about.

6. Lifestyle and Play

Play is not optional. It's medicine.

Ask:

- *What does joy look like in my day-to-day life?*
- *When do I feel most like myself?*
- *How can I make room for creativity, spontaneity, and fun—even now?*

Play brings color back into your world. It reminds your nervous system that life isn't just about doing and surviving—it's about being and living.

Create Your Vision Board

You can do this physically (with magazine cut-outs, drawings, or printed photos) or digitally. Choose images, words, and symbols that represent how you want to *feel* in these six areas, not just what you want to *have*.

Put your board somewhere you'll see it every day. Let it remind you of where you're heading, especially on the tough days.

**You're not visualizing fantasy—
you're visualizing possibility.**

Visualization

Close your eyes. Take a slow breath. Picture yourself six months, one year, or even five years from now—healthy, grounded, and living from your truth. What do you see? How do you feel when you wake up? Who's around you? What does your day look like?

Let yourself feel it fully—not as a wish, but as a reality you're already stepping into. Hold that vision. Then start acting like the person who's already there.

Your vision isn't about escaping where you are—it's about expanding who you are.

It's the bridge between the person you are and the person you're becoming.

Keep it close. Revisit it often. Adjust as you grow. This is a life plan. One built on peace, purpose, and possibility.

I can't keep count of the amount of times clients have sent emails and messages telling me how the vision and goals they set one or two years ago have all come true. In fact I just received a message last week from a past client Annette C from Australia.

She wrote:

> *Two years ago when I was in the program I took on the challenge to write about exactly how I wanted to have my life look like in the future. My story went on for pages. While trekking in Turkey, I realized that my life is exactly in line with my vision now. You had a saying Toby that said something like "invest in the things that will help you arrive at your vision," I guess that's what I am doing.*

Amazing right?

Now for context. Annette went from being totally bedbound, barely able to sit up in bed to trekking mountains for 26 days straight in Turkey. I messaged her back and asked her how far she actually walked. She replied between 350-400 km. (That's around 220-240 miles of walking over 26 days.) Unbelievable.

She set that vision when she was at her worst, she then did the actions and behaviors that helped her grow and progress from where she was to where she wanted to be. Now of course it wasn't easy. We worked together closely every single month to help her go from bedbound to living again. But I believe Annette's future vision helped her get through the hard times. It helped her stay accountable and helped her do whatever was required to get her life back one step at a time. You can do the same!

TAKEAWAYS

YOUR MINDSET DIRECTLY INFLUENCES YOUR RECOVERY: How you respond to challenges and setbacks act as opportunities for personal growth.

ACCEPT WHERE YOU ARE TODAY—NOT WHERE YOU USED TO BE. This is essential for restoring hope and creating forward momentum.

LET GO OF THE OLD TO BUILD THE NEW. Identity plays a major role in your healing. Let go of outdated identities and build new, empowered ones that support long-term progress.

QUESTIONS SHAPE OUTCOMES—shifting from fear-based or limiting questions to constructive, forward-focused ones. This opens the door to possibility and change.

RECOVERY INSPIRATION

Check out this free training on the 5 key traits of people who recover from CFS.

CHAPTER 8

FOOD IS FUEL

Food is fuel. Nutrition is a big part of your recovery toolkit. When people think about food they usually just think about something tasty to eat; however, food is much more than taste. Ancient philosophers and modern-day nutritionists can still agree centuries later, that there is no substitute for good nutrition. As Hippocrates said, "Let food be thy medicine and medicine be thy food."

Nutrition plays a foundational role in maintaining overall health and well-being, and how we eat, what we eat, and when we eat it matters. It influences every system in the body—from supporting immune function and hormonal balance to providing the energy required for cellular repair and cognitive performance. A well-balanced focus on nutritionally rich foods can reduce the risk of chronic diseases, improve mood, and enhance physical and mental resilience. I have seen the major role it plays in energy and emotions and I am a big advocate for learning to fuel your body without limiting your joy.

If Your Body Was a Ferrari

Imagine your body was a custom-made car of your choice, maybe a red Ferrari with a leather interior, or a slick Rolls Royce. Whatever you choose. How would you look after it? How would you fuel it? One thing is certain—you wouldn't put low-grade fuel in it. You'd look after it and maintain it with quality and care.

Your body can't be traded in like a car. It's the only vehicle you have for life. Best to fuel it well and not treat it like a trash can.

When it comes to recovery with CFS, nutrition becomes critical. With CFS, the body is in a state of stress, and nothing says "I'm safe" more than being completely satiated and well fed. If you think about this on a biological level, when we don't have food in our system, and we start to get hungry, the brain sends signals to the body that it is going into starvation mode.

What happens when a newborn baby gets hungry? They cry loudly. The longer they don't get fed, the louder they cry. But as soon as they get fed and the baby is satiated, what happens? The baby feels soothed and calms down.

This goes back to the hibernation theory, where the body shuts down to use less energy resources because it senses that there isn't enough energy to operate at a normal level.

Therefore, having proper nutrition during the recovery phase is an essential element to coaxing the body out of hibernation and ensuring there's enough energy to return to normal functioning. Think of animals that come out of hibernation. They are often weak and quickly need to find nourishing food and water to restore their bodies and gain energy after a long and intense hibernation period.

When your body or brain is under threat with a chronic illness, there's more likelihood that your brain signals detect danger. That means your nervous system gets triggered more easily than those without CFS. When you get hungry or are running on empty, you need to make sure that you are fueling your body regularly to stop it from panicking and going into survival mode. Make sense?

Plus, your brain and body are using more energy on a daily basis, trying to repair and heal from a chronic illness.

You have to fuel your body, so it gets the safety signal loud and clear.

Food is *fuel*.

Satiety is safety.

When you fuel your body regularly and consistently with the right food, you're going to be satiated for longer, your brain is going to work better, you're going to feel calmer, and you are going to feel safe. When well fed, your brain will send safety signals to your body that you are not going into starvation mode and that it's okay to use the energy it has stored up.

There is also a direct relationship between stress and food. Diet culture has skewed our sense of what is a healthy and nutritious diet and places far too much emphasis on maintaining a perfect diet. However, stressing about your food can actually be really counterproductive to your recovery. As always, a calm mindset will help you achieve more with less.

How McDonald's Helped Me Embrace Balance

Years ago, I had gut health issues. I tried everything—a vegan diet, carnivore diet, fasting, bone broth and keto. Nothing worked. I was so stressed out about the diet that the stress counteracted against any healthy diet that I was trying to maintain.

And of course, I didn't improve.

At the time I had no idea I was in this stressed state. I thought I was doing "everything right." The stress of getting things perfect and eating the right diet got in the way of me feeling relaxed and safe. I was behaving in a way that was completely at odds with embracing the healing powers of food.

My friend Charlie came over to visit me. He said, "Let's have pizza for dinner." I immediately replied, "I can't have pizza." I was doing a ketogenic diet at the time and although it wasn't working, I still held a shred of hope that it would be the magical cure.

Charlie looked at me, "Dude, you look like utter crap. You feel crap. You've been trying all these different diets for months and months and you still seem crap. You know what you need? You need McDonald's."

I was against the idea, still adamant that I had to stick to my diet.

"Dude, you're super stressed out. You just need to relax and eat a Big Mac. You need a burger and some chips; that'll fix your problems."

At this point, I was so over it, and since nothing was really working, I gave in. We got in the car and headed straight for the drive through. I didn't end up ordering a burger (I was still clinging on to some semblance of the diet), but I ordered the healthiest option I could—a chicken wrap with some chips. It was totally against the gut health protocol I'd been on for months, but heck, Charlie was right, I was undernourished and so stressed out, it wasn't doing me any good.

As the food arrived Charlie grinned and said, "You just need to enjoy your life, Toby. Stop stressing out about absolutely everything. Just take a bite. It's not gonna kill you."

I took a bite. My mouth did somersaults, "Oh, this tastes so good."

Charlie and I were laughing our heads off. He was like, "See, how much better do you feel now?"

"I actually do," I laughed as I crunched on fries.

And, more surprisingly, I was totally fine the next day too (of course!). There were no problems in my gut from that one chicken wrap and chips. And what that showed me is that ***it's not what you do, it's how you do it.***

Now, I'm not going to pretend that eating McDonald's is "healthy"; that's like me suggesting Ronald McDonald has the answer to CFS. But the point I want to make is this: **You don't need to have an all or nothing mentality to succeed**. And stressing about your food, even if it's super healthy, can be the thing keeping you stuck, stressed, and sick.

The stress and the pressure I put on myself to eat a perfect diet was inhibiting me from getting better. I was paralyzed by diet perfection. That day changed the game for me. I didn't have to have such a strong handle on, "I'm not allowed to eat this or I can't eat this." I eliminated stressful dieting the next day because I realized that what I was trying to do wasn't working anyway. In fact, I eliminated the word "diet" from my vocabulary; it wasn't working and was making me miserable.

Stressful dieting is *not* the remedy to good health.

I often suggest aiming for an 80/20 split. That 20% of "treat" food isn't going to do any detrimental damage, and what it does is allow you to enjoy your life and your diet and reap the benefits from the 80% that is within the boundaries of your healthy nutrition.

I'm a big believer in finding out what works for you and sticking to that. Remember the word body wisdom? That's what it is. Trusting your body wisdom and listening to it. The key is to tune into your body, ask it what it needs, and actually *listen*. Interpreting the message is also very important.

Listening to food cravings can be a valuable tool for understanding what your body may be lacking or needing. Cravings are not always random—they can be signals pointing toward specific nutritional deficiencies or emotional needs.

For example, if you find yourself craving sweets or chocolate, it might not just be a desire for sugar. Rather than immediately indulging or suppressing a craving, it can be helpful to pause and assess: *Am I tired? Stressed? Did I eat enough protein or healthy fats today? Is my craving for chocolate because I haven't eaten enough and I need a "quick hit?"*

By tuning into these signals with curiosity rather than judgment, we can start to respond more appropriately to what our bodies truly need—whether that's fruit, carbs, healthy fats or dairy (or maybe it really does just want the chocolate!).

And trust me, I love chocolate. Anyone who knows me, knows I *love* chocolate. Particularly dark chocolate. But you will never see me eat chocolate as a meal replacement. It will always be after a healthy fueled meal rich in protein, fats and good carbohydrates.

DON'T RUN ON EMPTY

If you think about it like a car, food and nutrition is to the body what petrol is to a car. When you've just filled up your car with a full tank of fuel, the car feels fuller and it's heavier, but it also runs more efficiently and speeds up quicker. When there's only a little bit of fuel left and you put your foot down, it's not picking up as fast and it's a little sluggish. The same rules apply for the human body. If you are running on empty, are you surprised that you can't get up and go?

Eating at the Right Time

We already touched on eating the right food at the right time to keep your circadian rhythm running correctly and helping you to sleep better, but it also helps your body distribute energy properly throughout the day. For instance, when you wake up in the morning and don't eat for the first couple of hours, you're running on empty. You've just fasted for 8–12 hours (or however long you sleep for) and if you try to avoid big meals a couple hours before bed like recommended, then that's even longer. Therefore, you need to replenish the tank and eat within the first hour or so of waking up, even if it's a little appetizer until you eat a full breakfast. That said, everyone's different so it's a matter of finding out what makes you feel the most energized and ready for the day.

The same principle applies to the rest of the day too, because if you have breakfast at 8am and then don't eat again until 3pm, you're essentially driving your car for as long as it gets you until you end up stranded in the middle of the road with no fuel. Instead, we want to provide multiple pit stops on the road trip that is your day, providing your body with constant sources of energy.

Josh Rubin from Real Food Gangstas once gave me a great analogy.

He said, "Toby, we want to treat your eating habits like we're keeping a fire going. In the mornings you start the fire with breakfast. This is where you put the foundation logs on. You have to set up your day with a good breakfast. This will start the fire well—high protein, good complex carbohydrates, and some healthy fats. You don't want to wait for the fire to burn out. You want to add logs (more food) to the already burning fire, and you continue to do this throughout the entire day."

Basically, he was saying—start the day off with a good foundational nutrient-dense breakfast within the first hour upon waking. And then don't wait to become hungry until you eat again. Keep fueling your brain and body throughout the day. Over time this will make a big difference.

When I start working with clients, many think they already eat healthily. But when I ask about their daily food intake and to give me a rundown on their average nutrition, their answers are usually the same. Something like this: "Yeah, I eat healthy most of the time. For breakfast I have tea or coffee and a piece of toast with jam on it."

I stop them right there. Toast ain't going to cut it as a "healthy breakfast." I then give some simple nutrition guidelines that fuels them rather than depletes them. So if you're having toast for breakfast. It ain't going to cut. Sorry, not sorry.

All jokes aside, everyone is different, and individual needs can vary based on factors like activity level, recovery stage, and personal preference. Most people benefit from eating every three to four hours, as this spacing allows for a steady supply of nutrients and energy, helping to prevent energy crashes from low blood sugar levels and we want to avoid that. Eating regularly also supports brain function and mood, as the brain relies on a consistent flow of protein, glucose and fats to function optimally. Skipping meals or going long periods without eating can lead to blood sugar dips, increased cortisol (stress hormone) levels, and disrupted digestion. A balanced pattern of three meals and one or two snacks daily can help keep the body fueled, reduce cravings, and promote sustained physical and mental performance.

EATING RIGHT

In my first book, *Chronic Fatigue Syndrome: a guide to recovery*, I worked with nutritionist, Steph Wearne and we included some helpful nutritional advice for CFS sufferers. I have included a summary here too.

We have all heard of protein, carbohydrates and fats, but it's important to know what they are, and what they actually do for you.

Protein

All tissues in our body are made and repaired with protein. Protein is responsible for growth and repair, as well as structure, production of vital organs, enzyme and hormone production, and nutrition for the immune system and transportation of nutrients.

Amino acids are the building blocks of protein. There are twenty amino acids the body requires for efficient function: eleven amino acids the body can make, and nine essential ones the body can't make—so we must get them from a food source.

Animal sources are a very rich source of protein, providing all the essential amino acids so they are referred to as complete sources of protein (see list below). Plant sources (apart from soy products) are not regarded as providing some of the essential amino acids and therefore need to be combined with other foods to provide a complete source of protein. Protein should take up one-quarter of our plate at every meal.

Animal sources:
- lean red meat
- poultry
- fish and shellfish
- dairy products
  (organic milk, yogurt
  and cheese)

Plant sources to combine:
- legumes and grains
- seeds, nuts, and grains

Carbohydrates

Carbohydrates are a primary source of fuel for our body. When we eat carbohydrates, they are broken down into glucose that the body uses for energy.

Carbohydrates should make up about half of our caloric intake for the day and approximately half of our food, depending on the individual's needs and energy outputs.

The type and amount of carbohydrates selected needs to be considered carefully, as when our blood glucose levels drop we experience tiredness, irritability, and mood highs and lows. The glycaemic index (GI) is a system that ranks carbohydrates depending on the rate of digestion and absorption (often referred to as simple carbohydrates) are digested and absorbed quickly, causing a spike in our blood glucose levels, whereas low GI foods (often referred to as complex carbohydrates) release glucose slowly and do not cause rapid rises in blood glucose levels. Lower GI foods give us more lasting energy.

The best types of carbohydrates to include in our diet are low GI complex and/or organic carbohydrates that are low in refined and milled flours. Fruit and vegetables, wholegrain and dairy products provide the best sources in this area. The following lists show types of carbohydrates we can use to take up one-quarter of our plate at every meal.

<table>
<tr><td colspan="2">Vegetables:</td><td>Wholegrains:</td></tr>
<tr><td>• sweet potato</td><td>• zucchini</td><td>• barley</td></tr>
<tr><td>• parsnip</td><td>• broccoli</td><td>• oats</td></tr>
<tr><td>• pumpkin</td><td>• cauliflower</td><td>• quinoa</td></tr>
<tr><td>• corn</td><td>• eggplant</td><td>• brown rice</td></tr>
<tr><td>• carrot</td><td>• green beans</td><td>• rye</td></tr>
</table>

In regards to wheat and grains, it's important to consider the impact gluten can have on your gut. For some people it isn't an issue but for others having gluten from certain breads, cereals, and pastas can wreak havoc with their gut. So, if you're experiencing bloating, inconsistent bowel movements or stomach pains, eliminating gluten from your diet could be a simple fix. It's best to trial which foods work best for you. Do what works. Stop doing what doesn't work. It will pay off.

Fats

There are certain healthy fats we can enjoy and others we should limit. The bad fats increase the LDL (low-density lipoprotein) cholesterol in our blood that contributes to plaque formation and the build-up of fatty materials on our blood vessel walls and greatly increases our risk of heart disease. The bad fats are known as saturated fats and trans fats. If we consume excess fat, it not only predisposes us to obesity and being overweight, it also increases our risk of other serious health conditions such as heart disease.

Healthy fats, otherwise known as monounsaturated fats and polyunsaturated fats, also increase the levels of HDL (good cholesterol) in the body, which removes LDL, leaving many other important functions in the body.

Cholesterol in foods has only a very small effect on cholesterol levels in your blood. It is the saturated fat in foods that affects your blood cholesterol level and should be kept to a minimum.

All fats should be consumed in small quantities in our diet, and the best sources of healthy fat for us to include in our diet are:

Healthy fats:

- egg yolks
- butter
- fatty animal cuts
- full fat yogurt
- nuts and seeds
- nut butters
- avocados
- olive oil
- fish/shell fish

Water

Many of us are under-hydrated without even realizing it. We can live weeks without food, but we can't survive without daily water. Our bodies are made up of approximately 60% water, so it's vital to our wellbeing and to know your individual needs for water intake as this can vary per day per person.

The following conditions require additional water intake:

- hot days
- excessive sweating
- heavy exercise
- alcohol consumption
- garden chores
- consumption of meat, eggs or salty foods
- fever

Vitamin food list

Nutrient	Function	Source
B vitamins	Promotes red blood cell production and energy levels.	Vegetables, wholegrain breads and cereals, legumes, nuts, seeds, meat, fish and eggs.
Omega 3 fatty acids	Reduces inflammation and boosts the body's ability to produce energy.	Fatty fish (salmon, sardines, mackerel), flaxseed oil, walnuts, chia seeds, soybeans.
Iron	Required for red blood cell production and oxygen carriage to cells.	Red meat, poultry, seafood, wholegrain cereals, spinach, legumes, dried fruits, nuts, seeds.
Magnesium	Energy production and metabolism, and reduces tiredness and fatigue.	Green leafy vegetables, nuts, seeds, whole grains, legumes, seafood.
Zinc	Antioxidant which can help fight the effects of harmful free radicals on damaged cells.	Meat, seafood, seeds, nuts, wholegrain cereals, beans, unrefined oil.

Intolerances and Allergies

Food intolerances and allergies are common with CFS, particularly wheat and dairy. It is worth eliminating these from your diet and reintroducing them after a few weeks to see if your symptoms improve. Bloating, gas and diarrhea are all signs of food intolerance. Here is a list of replacement foods you can use when eliminating wheat and dairy from your diet.

Wheat replacements:

- buckwheat
- millet
- quinoa
- brown rice

Dairy replacements:

- soy milk (non-GMO)
- oat milk
- rice milk
- almond milk
- coconut milk
- coconut yogurt

It's important to tune into your body and give it the food it responds best to. If you function better without wheat and dairy, do without it. If it's not a problem, it's not a problem. Remember treat your body like you would your favorite car. Care for it deeply and give it what it needs!

Staying nourished and adequately hydrated are the basics of good health, but it's important to have a balanced mindset too. **Take charge of your nutrition but don't let it take charge of you.** Remember eating to feel charged and energized isn't about restriction and stress, it's about wholesome and calm nourishment.

Nutrient-dense foods

One of the most important elements of nutrition is ensuring you're prioritizing nutrient dense foods. Nutrient-dense foods are sometimes called "superfoods" because they are packed with a high amount of vitamins, minerals, and other beneficial nutrients without containing too many calories, unhealthy fats, and added sugars. Essentially, these foods work really hard to build you a healthier body and immune system. These types of foods include avocado, fruit, black beans, broccoli, eggs, spinach, salmon, yogurt and potatoes. These foods will also keep you fuller for longer as they generally take longer to digest and therefore release energy equally over time.

For example, eating a whole orange will sustain you better and longer than drinking a glass of orange juice. This is because the orange contains fiber, which slows the release of sugar into your bloodstream and creates a steady release of energy (i.e., no big highs and crashes). Juice, on the other hand, is digested very quickly so it spikes your blood sugar without offering the same satiety or nutritional benefit.

Focusing on whole foods—such as fruits, vegetables, whole grains, lean proteins, and healthy fats—ensures you're getting the full range of nutrients your body needs to function properly. It's important to eat a variety of foods within each category, as different foods provide different nutrients. For instance, dark leafy greens are high in iron and calcium, while orange vegetables like carrots and sweet potatoes are rich in beta-carotene.

What can be tempting is to avoid certain food groups, and this has been the go-to for fad diets in the past twenty years. "Quit carbs!" "Quit sugar!" Avoid this and avoid that and you'll be healthier. However, avoiding entire food groups is unnecessary because our body needs them all. Carbohydrates, for instance, are the body's preferred source of energy, especially for the brain, and natural sugars in fruits and complex carbs in whole grains provide essential fuel and fiber. The key is choosing high-quality, minimally processed sources rather than cutting out food groups altogether. Balanced nutrition is about moderation, variety, and listening to your body's needs.

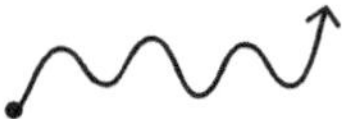

I once worked with a client called Cindy from the USA. Despite "doing all the right things" Cindy was stuck in her recovery.

We chatted on the phone and I asked her about her nutrition.

"It's great," she replied. "I eat vegan-friendly food. Toast for breakfast with a peanut butter spread, lots of fruit, salads and vegetables. I eat two to three times a day and it's generally pretty healthy."

"How do you feel after you eat? " I asked.

"Not great. My energy only lasts for around thirty minutes, then I feel depleted again."

I realized that Cindy was not eating enough protein for her daily intake. I asked her if she was open to trying animal protein for three months to see if it made a difference.

She said, "Toby, I have tried everything and nothing is working."

The only thing she hadn't tried was eating animal protein.

I reassured her there was no pressure, but I suspected that her strict diet may be limiting her body's ability to heal.

"Let's swap your toast and spread for a hearty breakfast of pasture raised eggs and some root vegetables. Then a smoothie as your snack with yogurt and collagen powder in it, some form of animal protein for lunch and dinner along with your fruit and vegetables."

Initially, Cindy was only open to eggs and fish. But it was a great start. I asked her to do what she felt comfortable with and reminded her that the whole goal was to give her brain and body the nutrients it needed to feel sustained for longer.

Cindy started to feel better within the first two weeks. More sustained energy, clearer mind, less brain fog, better mood and muscle recovery. Her sleep improved, she felt more stable, and because of that, she felt happier.

Within 3 months she felt so good, she completely changed her nutrition plan to more animal protein like beef, chicken, and more seafood.

Cindy went on to fully recover, not only because of the nutrition, but because it was one of the missing pieces to her recovery puzzle.

Whichever approach you take when it comes to your food, do what works, stop doing what doesn't. There are two things I want you to remember:

1. Food is fuel.
2. Enjoy what you eat. It's one of life's pleasures.

TAKEAWAYS

FOOD IS FUEL: Food is much more than just a means to satisfy hunger or taste buds—it's essential for supporting overall health, immune function, and mental performance. What we eat, how we eat, and when we eat significantly impact our well-being, with a balanced diet reducing the risk of chronic diseases and boosting physical and mental resilience.

NUTRITION IS PART OF YOUR RECOVERY TOOLKIT: Nutrition plays an especially critical role when recovering from CFS, as proper fuel helps the body escape its survival mode. Consistent, nourishing meals reassure the brain that there's no need for the body to conserve energy, aiding in recovery and reducing stress triggers from hunger.

EMBRACE BALANCE: After struggling with gut health and extreme dieting, I realized that stressing over perfect eating habits hindered my healing. A moment of embracing balance— eating a fast-food meal—taught me that it's not about perfection but how we approach food. Adopting a more relaxed mindset helped me feel better and focus on long-term health.

DON'T RUN ON EMPTY: Just like a car needs a full tank to run efficiently, our bodies need constant nourishment. Regular meals—ideally every 3–4 hours—ensure we don't run on empty, providing consistent energy and supporting brain function. This routine prevents energy crashes and stress while helping with physical and mental performance.

RECOVERY INSPIRATION

Check out these videos on nutrition and why food matters.

CHAPTER 9

Movement

How can you live your best life if you don't have the strength and stamina to do things? Shopping, lifting up the kettle to pour tea, driving a car, making love with your partner, walking around the park, holding a baby, or taking the dog for a walk, *all* require strength and stamina.

STRENGTH IS LIFE

Movement is often an overlooked aspect of recovery, but it's one of the most vital.

It's not as simple as "doing exercise" because the wrong movement or too much at the wrong time can make you feel worse.

Movement and exercise need a nuanced approach depending on what stage of recovery you are in. It's not as generic as graded exercise therapy which is outdated and often over-prescribed and often makes people feel worse.

This chapter is about building strength so you have a solid foundation to spring from. It's not about 'working out' or 'exercising' like you used to know it. I won't be talking about bulging biceps, six-packs, or pushing yourself beyond your means. I will be talking about strength as your life force, strength that helps you feel restored, balanced, and well.

We will go together step by step.

"Tiptoe if you must, but take a step."
—Naeem Callaway

Strength is not something you feel you have when going through CFS, it can feel almost impossible to have any. The good news is that over time you can rehabilitate your brain and body and build strength back into your body. And that's what you need to do in order to live your best life.

Movement is critically important. I know, I know—you are told that there are so many things to focus on in recovery, and here is yet another. But if you think about post-recovery and life itself, you are required to move every single day, so it's important you have the strength to do so.

Strength Is the Foundation for Life

One of the biggest problems with chronic fatigue syndrome is the deconditioning of the body. You don't have the energy to do what you used to be able to do, and so you lose muscle mass, usually gain fat or become severely underweight and lose condition altogether. Science also backs this, revealing that people with CFS did experience low exercise capacity, deconditioning of the body, and felt weaker than those merely unfit or sedentary.[6]

Therefore, reconditioning your body appropriately is an integral step of recovery. The more muscle mass you have, the more energy is stored in your body. The more energy you have, the better you can live and enjoy life.

There are two ways to build strength. One is through daily-life function and the other is through structured, intentional movement. In this chapter, I am going to break down how and when to implement movement into your recovery so it helps you get stronger without feeling worse.

This isn't just about recovery. Movement is just as important when you're healthy and it's not something you stop when you've recovered. It's a lifelong thing as there are so many benefits to it. Provided it's the right amount and appropriate for where you are, it can be great for your mindset and good for your physical strength and building your capacity. But it also does a lot of wonderful things with your body and brain too! Not only does it improve your overall physical health, it reduces the risk of chronic diseases, enhances mood, reduces stress and anxiety and promotes better sleep.

Despite this, it's common for the word *exercise* to not go hand-in-hand with CFS and this is for a few reasons. We often perceive exercise as pushing our body to the limits—the old "no pain, no gain" philosophy. Exercise is also often wrongly prescribed by health professionals to patients with CFS, as they don't actually understand CFS and end up over prescribing exercise too early because the patient "doesn't look sick." The person then feels like they need to "push through," but they of course end up crashing and feeling worse than they did before. There's even a medical term for this—post-exertional malaise (PEM)—which is basically a fancy word for the worsening of symptoms following any basic physical or mental exertion. We all know that feeling.

But we must always remember that recovery isn't linear and our well-being and energy levels vary day to day. We aren't required to "do it all" to make progress. We need to factor in poor quality sleep, lack of quality nutrition, stress, and colds and flus, and make sure we're not pushing the boundaries of our baseline.

This is why we don't use the word exercise here at CFS Health and instead we refer to it as "appropriate restorative movement." We teach our clients to know their body so well that they can adapt their movement approach on any given day based on how they feel. The great thing about this is that it creates more consistent and appropriate movement for the client's level and therefore allows the brain and body to adapt appropriately to the stimulus without feeling worse. The result? Increases in strength, capacity and health.

I like to use the word "movement" rather than exercise because movement is so multifaceted. It's broad. There's no bad connotation that comes with it. Even so, I think there's a lot of fear for some people about movement because most movement or exercise programs aren't appropriate for where they are right now, especially if you are in the first stage of recovery in the restore zone. You may be fighting off a virus, sleeping 15–16 hours a day, and you're exhausted. Overdoing it with movement can be the opposite of useful. Slow and steady wins the race.

The mistake I made, that I never let a client make.
As I got better from CFS, I decided to jump back into playing basketball. I was feeling better but hadn't done much strength and conditioning training at the level playing basketball needed. At the time I didn't realize this.

So when the referee blew the whistle and threw the ball in the air to start the game, I was pumped.

Three short minutes later, I went up for a rebound, and as I was coming down (over the top of a player from the other team), my left arm went over his body and my shoulder was dislocated. To say it was painful is an understatement.

I went for emergency surgery the next day. I needed a full shoulder reconstruction. It took an entire year of rehab to return to full strength and functionally in that arm.

Although I was recovered from CFS, my body wasn't fully prepared and conditioned to be back at high level sport. It was one of the most impactful lessons I took into my career helping others recover from CFS.

I worked with a lot of people who wanted to get back into sports, and it was through my own personal experience, training and duty of care, to make sure no one else went through a similar injury experience. I would make sure my clients were ready and conditioned *before* they entered back into any sports or physical endeavors.

For example, client Steph Ryan, who I mentioned earlier in the book. Before CFS she was a gun netball player. She loved the game so much. CFS not only sidelined her health, it sidelined her passion. When she first came to me she was suffering so badly that she could barely walk.

Her dream goal was to one day get back to playing netball. Now of course this didn't happen overnight. But we had a goal… and over time, as we got her baseline right and slowly introduced restorative movement into her program, we built up her capacity in an appropriate way. We slowly incorporated netball skills and drills into her movement plan so she could get the feel of netball again on a consistent basis. Six to twelve months later she was a different person. Healthy and eager to keep moving her life forward.

And then the time came. She was ready to get back to netball.

But it was important to not throw her in the deep end, but to have a progressive plan that eased her into playing netball at a competitive level.

Initially it was just a few minutes of game time. Then we increased the time on the court each week until she progressed to the four quarters of a netball game.

This meant her body and brain were strong enough to handle the load and no injuries happened as a result.

Today, ten years later, Steph is the exercise physiologist and specialized movement coach at CFS Health and she helps people make the return to healthy movement.

She knows through lived experience and her professional career how important it is to get this right. She also knows that if you want to return to hiking, then you will need strong ankles. If you love fishing, you will need strong wrists for casting out. If you want to return to dancing, you will need a strong body from the ground up. Equally, if you're a painter or musician, you will need to do resistance training for strong arms and hands. There are so many different reasons why we move our bodies and it's important that you find your why. Find what you love and return to it in a planned way.

In fact, we designed our entire restorative movement program for our members to help them recondition their bodies appropriately from where they are at now to where they want to be. There are 12 levels inside our movement mastery program and they cover all stages of recovery because it's important to have a tiered and monitored approach to movement over time.

For some added inspiration, watch Steph's full recovery success story here:

FIND YOUR WHY

Why do you want to move your body? Maybe you have an overarching goal that you want to focus on, like going on a hike. Maybe you want to be able to go on that holiday you had planned. What is it for you? What is your why? Why do you want to get stronger?

If we have something driving us to move, we're more likely to do it, we're more likely to enjoy it, and we can see that goal at the end. For many people, they want to move their body because it helps them get their life back. It's an overall view, as opposed to having a specific reason.

While we are young and healthy, we can get away without strength training; however, it becomes clear when we start to get older how this lack of movement affects us. In our forties and fifties, we'll start to slow down and may not feel as strong or as flexible as before. In our sixties, this could mean not being able to walk for more than thirty minutes or picking up a grandchild. Even further on, we may struggle to tie our shoelaces, get off the toilet, and lift medium-heavy items. Training for strength and flexibility protects our independence and quality of life, so do it for you now, do it for your future self, do it for your elderly self, and do it for your family and friends. Do it for the goals and dreams you eventually want to actualize.

For people with CFS specifically, being strong means we can tolerate a lot more. We essentially live the life we want to live, and that's what we want to aim for.

If you don't have a goal, it's harder to be consistent with it. You'll start for two weeks and then your motivation and commitment will run out. So write it down now.

Why do I want to be strong?
Why does being strong matter to me?

____

____

____

____

What freedom will it give me?
Why does this matter to me?

____

____

____

____

THE DIFFERENT TYPES
OF MOVEMENT

Daily Functional Movement

If you are reading this thinking, *Oh, but I can't move at all. I have zero fitness.*

Well, you're here right now, holding a book in your hands, so you *can* move. It all counts. Sitting up in bed can count as movement, looking at a screen or moving your head can count as movement. Even moving your feet and hands in bed counts.

I've had people join me on a call and say, "I'm not moving yet." I ask them what they did that day and often they'll say, "I got out of bed, I went to the toilet, I showered and I dressed myself." That sounds like movement to me.

If you are in your room and you spend a lot of time there, just moving from one space to another can also be really beneficial in the early stages of recovery. That is all still classified as movement, and this is what we call "daily functional movement." It's anything you need to do to live your life on a day-to-day basis—even something as simple as brushing your teeth and making a cup of tea!

Structured Movement

Then there is structured movement and that's what you schedule in. It's got a time and a place, a specific modality of training and you're going to tick it off for the day. It could be anything from restorative strength movements, yoga, Pilates, walking/biking, rowing or even stretching. Even if it's for one minute or ten minutes or more, it all counts and it's all important. If you are choosing to do a specific modality of movement to increase strength, stamina and fitness, it falls under the category of structured movement.

Aerobic / Cardiovascular Movement

Aerobic movement, also known as cardiovascular movement or

cardio, includes repetitive, steady motions that engage the large muscle groups. Examples include walking, running, hiking, cycling, and swimming. There are a plethora of benefits to this type of movement, including weight management, strengthening of the heart, lungs and circulatory system, reduction in risk of chronic diseases, boosted mood, increased stamina, and a stronger immune system. For people with CFS, incremental activity (slowly building up the level and duration of activity) has shown to improve muscle strength, cardiovascular endurance and reduce symptoms. It will also reduce overall body or muscular fatigue. When you are out walking (to limits appropriate to your baseline), you are gaining energy. Movement can produce energy if done appropriately. Don't worry, you don't have to keep overdoing it and feel worse. I will show you a framework that we give all our members that helps stop the ups and downs, decreases the likelihood of PEM, and helps you feel better, not worse.

Strength Training

Over time, you will be ready for a structured type of movement called strength training, and there's a lot of research that proves the combination of strength training and cardio provides great outcomes for people with chronic conditions. It involves using your body weight or weights to conduct a push or pull movement, like squats and pushups. It can also be stationary and involve endurance of muscles by holding a position, like planks and wall sits.

These actions build muscle and stamina, but just because it's called strength training doesn't mean it involves pushing yourself beyond your limits or lifting super heavy weights. In the early days, this could be as simple as lifting a pillow in bed. Resistance training is about building strength and stamina from where you are at right now. I had a client whose first strength exercise was sitting up in bed. She used to lay down all the time, so we started getting her to sit up regularly throughout the day. Her second strength training exercise was doing a pillow pushup. She was laying on her back and she just held the pillow and pushed it up and down. It was a really light pillow, but it was still super helpful for her, because it was appropriate for her capacity. Essentially, she was activating her muscles and giving them a purpose. It's a way of saying to the muscles, "Hey, can you wake up? I want you to switch on." Over time and with consistency, strength builds. And then higher outputs of capacity happen without feeling worse.

The benefits of strength training range from an increase in muscular strength to improved bone density and cardiovascular health, lower risk of chronic disease, boosted metabolism and improved sleep, flexibility, mobility, mood and overall well-being.

There is also improvement in your posture. When you are fatigued, posture isn't great as you're often sitting or lying for long periods and you adapt to a position where your shoulders roll forward. That's really normal. But the issue is the muscles along the front become really short and tight and the muscles along our back become really long and weak.

Using strength training can recondition those muscles and make them stronger, which will in turn pull your shoulders back into a good position.

Inside our online recovery program we highly recommend our 12 level restorative movement program because it's safe, effective and designed specifically for people with CFS. It's so flexible that you can start it from your home, or even your bed if you're on the lower end of capacity. It's all about reconditioning your body so you can do what you want to do, when you want to do it.

When you figure out which movement you like and to what level makes you feel good, it is a real turning point in your recovery.

What about Graded Exercise Therapy (GET)?

I know you may be thinking - *Isn't this gradual movement philosophy just graded exercise therapy?* No, it's not. Let me explain…

Graded exercise therapy (GET) is an outdated and fixed exercise methodology that doesn't take into account the patient's day-to-day symptoms and other lifestyle factors. It's usually conducted in a supervised manner by a physiotherapist or exercise therapist with the idea to reverse deconditioning. It's often over-prescribed and relies on a fixed exercise structure regardless of how the individual is feeling day to day. GET is now widely discouraged for CFS because it does not account for post-exertional malaise (PEM) and can lead to symptom exacerbation if wrongly prescribed.

This is why I only encourage using a Flexible Movement Framework. A flexible daily approach is required so that the person with CFS can adapt their movement according to their life. For example, adapting movement during illness or a stressful period in life is essential. At CFS Health we teach our members how to tune into their bodies and stop overdoing things. How to gradually build up capacity in a flexible way that takes the whole person and their lifestyle and what they're going through into account.

Flexible Movement Framework

Remaining flexible but still progressing in your movement happens in stages. But here's one ultra easy way to ensure you can still enjoy movement without pushing beyond your capacity.

It's all about your RPE.

RPE = rate of perceived exertion.

Using this flexible framework I'm about to show you is one surefire way to ensure you can stay in the "sweet spot" of your movement progression.

You can use this for:

- physical activity output
- cognitive activity output
- energy out activities (or any output for that matter).

It's incredibly useful and versatile.

We use the RPE scale of 0-10.

0 = no effort whatsoever.

As the numbers go up, the more effort is required in terms of output. 10 = absolute maximum effort.

Now we wouldn't want anyone recovering from CFS, especially in stage 1 and 2 of recovery, to go even close to a 10/10 on the RPE scale of effort.

When members start with us, we help them establish their appropriate baseline first. It's imperative to stop the push-crash cycle. We use the RPE scale to make sure they don't overdo it.

For most cases, I recommend starting out with activities that do not exceed 3-4 on the RPE scale. Meaning that any activity does not exceed a 3 or 4 exertion out of 10. This ensures the client is doing what is appropriate and they will be able to maintain their baseline and therefore progress responsibly.

The great thing about using the RPE scale is that over time, as you get better, you can do more without feeling worse. So you can do things with more effort and feel fine after. The other cool thing is as you get stronger, what used to be a 5/10 effort is only now a 2/10 effort. Which means your capacity is higher and you can do more in a day with much more ease.

The other great thing about RPE is that it's flexible. Especially as you get better. You can use the RPE scale to do what's right for you on any given day. Some days you may feel like doing less because you didn't sleep well the night before.

So you can back down your activities from a 6/10 to a 3/10 and do what is right for you at any given moment. This is what we call body wisdom.

In a world that glorifies punishing or pushing your body into pain and exhaustion, pulling back can feel challenging. This can be hard at first but once you do it, you will not look back. This flexible approach is something you carry with you for the rest of your life even when you're healthy and living fully again.

As I said before, the RPE scale can be used in all areas of life to help you determine and navigate your energy output, not just physically but cognitively and emotionally too.

Take a Long-Term View

Over time, as you implement flexible movement appropriately for you and you prioritize consistency over intensity, your resting heart rate will drop and your strength and stamina will increase. There will be bumps in the road, and that's fine. That's life. But when you do the right kinds of movement that work for you and you stick with it, what was once hard becomes easy.

The most important thing about choosing which type of movement to do is to make sure you enjoy it. If there is a certain movement modality that you really do not enjoy, take it off the list right now. You don't have to do everything and you should never do something you don't want to do or do something you don't feel comfortable doing, as we need to have a positive relationship with the movement we do.

The biggest factor of success when it comes to sticking to a movement routine is joy. As neuromuscular therapist Carol Welch-Baril said, " Movement is a medicine for creating change in a person's physical, emotional, and mental states."

But I will say with structured restorative movement, you may not feel heaps of "joy" doing it, but what it gives you in the long run will bring so much joy as you get stronger and healthier. So see it as a benefit not as a drawback.

Should You Make a Habit of Stretching?

A lot of people I work with love yoga and stretching. Some people ask me if they should be stretching during recovery and the answer is simple: If it feels good for you and you enjoy it, do it. If you don't get a good response or you're not enjoying it, don't do it. Simple as that.

That said, I want to tell you about some of the benefits of stretching: it improves our range of motion, can help reduce muscle pain, helps blood circulation, improves our posture and helps release stress. Also, if we are focusing on our breath during stretching or while doing yoga, it can be a form of active meditation, which is helpful for both our body and mind.

Movement Snacking

If doing any type of structured movement feels overwhelming for you, you can try to dip your toes in using the "movement snacking" method. It's exactly what it sounds like: doing mini sessions or mini movements at multiple points during the day, just as you would snack on food between meals.

Depending on what stage you're at, those mini movements might be standing up from the couch, sitting back down, standing back up, and then sitting back down periodically while watching TV. Or doing a wall pushup against the kitchen wall as you get some food. No matter how small, you've added in more movement into that particular moment of your day. You might add these throughout your routine so that even if you're not ready for bigger sections of structured movement, you're still working towards that goal in achievable chunks. You are allowing your body to rest and adapt to how you are feeling rather than doing one big session when you're first starting with movement. Movement snacking can mean less fatigue because you've not done it in one big go. Give it a try if that feels more comfortable for you.

We give our clients the flexibility to do either movement snacking or more structured movement sessions depending on what works for them. They obviously have specific movements inside the program that help recondition their body, but how they do it is up to them. Whether it be snacking movements or more structured sessions. The key is to start appropriately for where you are.

RAFF

When Raff first reached out to me, she had minimal movement in her day. She spent most of her days in bed. So we began her movement program right there, in bed.

We started with one chin tuck that she would hold for three seconds. She had a lot of upper back pain, so this movement was targeted at relieving the tension. After a few days of doing one chin tuck, she added in two or three into her day. She was soon able to add in a secondary exercise, which was an iso-metric quad squeeze that was aimed at activating her muscles again. She was still in bed most of the time when she was doing this, she would lay in bed and squeeze her quad muscle for three seconds.

Raff did that consistently for about two or three weeks, and then she did two lots of quad squeezes, then three lots of them, and then she added in a third exercise. She was exercise-snacking throughout her days. Naturally, this depended a lot on her capac-ity and how she was feeling on a particular day.

Raff took her journey slowly but surely and eventually her movement increased to getting out of bed and starting some daily functional movement around the house.

From there, Raff progressed into our specific restrengthening program and built her strength and stamina up over time. She did the same for her walking too. Raff built up her capacity so much during her first year that she was able to travel to the ski slopes with her family and ski without soreness or fatigue.

Nowadays, you wouldn't recognize her. Raff is skiing, walking and bike riding—she loves movement. She's always smiling and on the go. Raff has gone from bedridden to bouncing around living her best life.

But Raff's story isn't isolated. One report revealed that around **25% of people with CFS become housebound or bedbound.** [7] So how can we expect recovery to happen in gyms and outside the home? We can't! Recovery must begin wherever the person can; that could be in the bed or in the home first. And often it is.

MOVEMENT THROUGH THE STAGES OF RECOVERY

As we know, doing the right things at the right time will get the right results. When it comes to movement, this couldn't be any more paramount to recovery. Pushing ourselves to do more physically is only going to lead to burnout, fatigue, and potentially injury, the exact same way it would if a healthy person ran twenty miles without any training. No matter which stage you're in, I want you to be honest with yourself about it and make sure you've fully reached acceptance on what your baseline is. Only then can you start to build up and make physical (and cognitive) progress toward your recovery.

Movement in Stage 1: the restore stage.

The first stage of CFS is the acute phase of suffering—you're struggling with symptoms and you're feeling totally exhausted. It's usually at these initial stages when you might have a virus, you are actively going through a heavy infection, you might have come out of a prolonged period of stress or the initial stage of CFS.

In this time, I would *not* recommend structured movement at all, because you don't need to expend any more energy than you currently have. Instead, we need to put energy back in and we can do this by:

- restorative breathing
- restorative movement
- daily functional movement

Use your daily activities as movement and start to build your capacity this way. You'll find that over time your daily functional movement around the house will expand and you'll slowly be able to do more. Simply going outside, watering the plants, going to the bathroom, sitting up for breakfast, lunch and dinner, going from the bed to the couch, sitting up for longer, standing up for longer, all these things add up if you do them consistently over time.

You will know that you're ready for the next stage only when you are managing daily functional movement without continual exhaustion and malaise. You will feel an improvement in your capacity to do home tasks and your sleep and general wellbeing will be consistent.

Now, as you feel able, you can implement a very small structured movement routine appropriate for where you're at. We would call these micro- sessions, rather than macro-structured sessions. Meaning they are small, appropriate and doable. This would typically start from your bed or bedroom floor. Over time, as you get stronger, you will be able to do more and slowly expand your daily function and structured movement sessions.

Movement in Stage 2: the restrengthen stage.

This stage is where you come out of the acute stage of suffering and your energy is starting to come to the body, but it's like your brain doesn't know what to do with it. Feeling tired and wired in this stage can be normal. In this stage, we can work toward doing more structured movement, but still very restorative. This can start with "movement snacking" here, doing really small but purposeful movements throughout the day that will build your capacity.

Once you're feeling strong from that you can move on to bigger macro movement sessions that incorporate major muscle groups of the body.

Of course based on your goals, you will select specific movement modalities that will help you achieve them. Say you want to get back to hiking, it makes sense to incorporate a walking program and build up over time, along with the restorative restrengthening to maintain good muscle condition and overall strength and capacity.

In regards to your progress, you want to make sure you maintain your current capacity and movement regime for a minimum two to four weeks consistently so the body can adapt appropriately before adding more. However, remember that your movement progress is not linear and that it's okay to adapt on a day-to-day basis.

Using the RPE scale will help you adapt accordingly. On some days it will be a little less, other days it can be a little more.

Once you have maintained your progress, you can move to a new level. You may add more repetitions per movement or more sets, or both depending on where you are at. If it's cardiovascular, you can progress by seconds/minutes or intensity. Don't worry I cover progress on a deep level in the next chapter.

Remember you don't want to go from zero to hero. Small increments done consistently over time work best. You never want to force progress, but rather feel pulled to naturally do more over time. This is a true sign of progress.

If you have to pull back on movement at times, this is not a failure—it's a sign that you are getting to know your body and listening to it. This is an excellent skill. If what you are doing is compromising your entire week or even your whole day; it's too much for where you're at right now and it's more productive to scale it down.

Movement in Stage 3: the integration phase.
As you integrate back into life, your strength and capacity will be increased and your immune system is better, so that means you can handle more physiologically. Therefore, you can start doing more macro sessions, which is the more progressed training from smaller sessions. This is where you will be doing 20, 30, 40 minutes or even longer (if it's aligned with your goals and dreams).

You will know you're ready for this because you have progressed appropriately all the way along your journey and you are naturally feeling pulled to do more and you have the strength/capacity to do so. This is when you will be moving towards more life movement goals, whether that be hiking, dance classes, yoga/pilates classes, skiing, snowboarding, surfing, or cycling. The choice is yours.

Movement-wise, make sure you're doing the compound movements: so we're targeting all our multi-joint movement sessions, so think about hips, knees, arms and back. Multi-joint is where we are using multiple joints in the movement. Single joint exercises, they're good, that would be more like a bicep curl and a tricep pushdown kind of thing, but they're not targeting multiple muscles in one movement.

Multi-joint movements are things like squats or lunges or bench press/ rows.

In stage 3 you will be doing more healthy movement routines or at least building towards them so you can eventually do whatever you would like.

RECAP OF RECOVERY

Once you know where you are on the roadmap of recovery, either stage 1, 2 or 3, you can build a routine that suits you, stay consistent, build on it, and then get to the next level. It's not overnight. Nothing is.

Stage 1—focus on building functionality around the house.

Stage 2—you can start restorative movement but keep the intensity low, so it's easy, doable, and it feels good.

Stage 3—you can start to do more macro sessions that are aligned with your life movement goals. As you get better, you can do more as your body adjusts.

If you are thinking, *What's the quick fix? Tell me the secret.* I just told you the secret:

Start now from wherever you are and build. Consistency over intensity is the secret. Start with the minimum effective dose of movement for you with where you are at and build from there.

If you do all this properly and you start at the appropriate level, PEM should not exist. You can avoid these types of flare ups when you do the appropriate amount. You may experience DOMS, but not post-exertion malaise.

Let me explain.

What Is a Micro-Tear?

A lot of people don't realize that when doing strength training, micro tears occur in the muscle and then the body repairs them to make them stronger and bigger than before. The process is called hypertrophy, and it's where DOMs (delayed onset muscle soreness) comes into play.

We create micro tears when we do movement, so this is why it's important to have a gradual and appropriate approach. If you go too hard or lift too heavy, those tears will get bigger and may lead to injury. It's best to avoid going too hard and getting to that level of output because you can get injured and it's an unreasonable level to maintain.

Before I got chronic fatigue syndrome as a teenager, I used to think that when I was doing my bicep curls, my biceps were literally growing as I did the exercise. And so I was doing bicep curls and thinking, *Oh my God, they're growing.* As I learned exercise science, I realized that muscle growth doesn't happen when you are doing the movement. It happens in the rest and repair stage after movement. You'll train and create micro tears, and then in the next 24–48 hours, with adequate sleep, nutrition, rest and recovery, your body repairs that muscle and adapts appropriately to the new stimulus.

This is why all the elements, sleep, nutrition/hydration and movement, are so important, because each one feeds into the next and it creates a cycle of well-being.

Consistency over intensity is the main goal with strength training and all other forms of movement, but that doesn't mean you have to do it every day. Especially in the later stages of 2 and 3 because your overall output is higher you can actually have more days off in between as rest/repair days. If you are in stage 1 or 2 and doing micro sessions every day (or close to every day) that's okay because they are smaller sessions and you're keeping your overall energy output low on the RPE scale. This ensures it's safe and effective.

Once you're at this stage of movement, three strength sessions coupled with regular cardio and rest days is an ideal routine. Again it all depends on your personal goals and what you are working towards.

Symptom Versus Muscular Fatigue

Speaking of DOMs, we need to know what is considered a "good sore" and a "bad sore." DOMS (delayed-onset muscle soreness) is what every single healthy human being gets after training, depending on the load that they do. When done at a standard level, it can last between 24–48 hours. If you haven't done a Pilates class for a long time and you go do one, I can almost guarantee that you will be sore later in the week. The worst day for DOMS is usually the second day, so if you are a little bit sore on day one and then you wake up on day two and you're finding it sore to walk up the stairs or sit on the toilet, that's totally normal.

We can actually decrease the amount of DOMS you experience by decreasing the overall intensity and output of your movement sessions, this is why we get our clients to use the RPE scale and set an appropriate level first so they don't experience much soreness or fatigue at all. You are sore enough with CFS. The point isn't to make you sorer. It's to move and recondition your body without feeling any worse than you currently do.

The difference between appropriate muscular fatigue and CFS symptom soreness is very simple. It's when it is no longer considered "sore" around the specific muscle groups you used and instead it moves into a widespread pain and soreness across the entire body. This is when we get the whole-body aches and it lasts more than 48 hours (if it does last for more than 48 hours but is improving and doesn't stop you from doing everyday things, then this is still normal). It doesn't feel good. We know something is off. Maybe some of your symptoms are popping back up and you don't have the strength to do another session a few days later. Or you're not waking up consistently each day with the same energy levels and you're slowly getting worse in some areas.

That's moving into post-exertion malaise (PEM) and it's not smart for recovery. It can delay progress and as it often involves pain, it means you may skip a session or two simply because you're so sore. A slow but steady approach will get you better results and help progress faster.

The other indicator that you're doing too much is that your symptoms come on during the activity or soon thereafter. Remember, appropriate muscular fatigue in the specific muscles you are using is fine, it's the inappropriate symptoms that come up during or after activity that you don't want.

You are better off underdoing it initially rather than overdoing it. A less is more approach will set you up well. I call this the minimum effective dose.

On the other side of things, if you don't get DOMS, does it mean you haven't done enough? No. It means your body is probably already adapted to it or it's within your baseline, and that's not a bad thing. It might mean at some point you need to progress, but your body is moving and it knows what it's doing or what's required, so it doesn't need to give you that response. Because you are going through recovery and particularly if you are in stages 1 or 2, you want to minimize DOMS initially as you get started. As you progress of course you can do more and handle more DOMS. Stage 3 is where you can do a lot more and where you can progress a lot faster. Because your muscles can adapt to more stimulus.

There are what I call "progress weeks" and "maintenance months." It's important to have periods where you maintain where you're at, even if it feels easy. That's a good thing. You don't necessarily want to aim for soreness as the outcome of every session and it's not a prerequisite for building up strength. I've said it many times before, but I'll say it again: consistency over intensity!

Replenish and Recover

There are many ways to recover while doing movement training. You might eat something high in protein (this helps your body to repair those micro tears more efficiently), do magnesium or Epsom salt baths (reduces soreness) or stick your legs up on the wall (helps with blood flow). These are all really good for soothing your muscles after a big session.

For those smaller sessions or even for the functional daily movement, we can also do rituals that help us to recover. For instance, if you catch public transport to go grocery shopping, this can be very stimulating and exhausting. To avoid getting exhausted in the first place, you could try inserting mini recharge points along your journey, like sitting on a park bench in silence for ten minutes after getting off the train/bus and before going into the store. When you get home, you might then like to wind down by eating a healthy snack, having a cup of tea, closing your eyes and listening to music, or doing a restorative breathing exercise.

The point is that after doing any form of movement or "energy out" activity, it is totally okay (and recommended) to follow it up with something that recharges your battery. We can build a set of activities that we know work for us, and this is what I call our "recharge pack." Whatever is part of your recharge package is completely up to you. Find what works for you. It's creating a space where you can recharge before you go and do your next thing and this is far more productive than trying to move on to the next "energy out" activity with an empty battery. We shouldn't have to wait for fatigue or for our body to tell us that we need to slow down, but we're going to be pro-active and charge it before it reaches zero.

Activities that could be included in your energy pack might be:

1. **Legs-up-the-wall pose (Viparita Karani):** A gentle inversion that helps improve circulation, reduce swelling, and promote relaxation. (Lay on your back on the floor, elevate your legs against a wall or a couch, stretch your legs ideally or keep them slightly bent, lay there and relax for five or ten minutes. Make sure you don't get up too quick, sit against the wall or couch before you stand up.)

2. **Listening to calming music or nature sounds:** Helps soothe the nervous system and create a peaceful mental space.

3. **Epsom salt or magnesium baths:** Relieves muscle tension and supports the nervous system—especially good after physical activity.

4. **Restorative breathing or guided meditation/ Yoga Nidra:** Even 3–5 minutes can reset the body and calm an overactive stress response.

5. **Sipping herbal tea (like chamomile, ginger, or lemon balm):** Hydrating and comforting, helps you pause and be present.

6. **Short nature break (sit outside or near a window):** Being in or viewing nature can reduce fatigue, lower stress, and improve mental clarity.

7. **Mindless entertainment (light comedy, soothing podcasts):** Provides mental rest and a mood boost without taxing cognitive energy.

8. **Eating a nutrient-dense snack:** Something easy to digest, that has a mix of protein, complex carbohydrates and healthy fats.

9. **Aromatherapy (lavender, eucalyptus, peppermint oil):** Can support relaxation or gentle stimulation depending on your needs.

10. **Creative expression (art, gentle journaling, sketching, knitting):** Activities that don't require structure or goals but feel satisfying.

11. **Progressive muscle relaxation**: Guides your attention inward and helps release tension you may not realize you're holding.
12. **Hydration with electrolytes:** Supports energy production and blood volume regulation.
13. **10-minute silent break (no screens, noise, or light)**: Acts like a "mental nap" and can be surprisingly restorative.

A WORD ON FEAR

I think everyone goes through a degree of fear at some stage in their recovery, particularly if something hasn't worked or there's been a setback. Fear is a normal response for the brain and the body, as it almost goes into flight-or-fight mode and it says, "You know what? I don't want to do that anymore. It didn't feel good."

When this happens, the first question to ask is, "Am I safe?" At the end of the day, we're generally pretty safe, but if you don't feel safe, is there a way to feel more safe? Is it by being in an environment that feels safer to you? Is it by playing some music that's calming? How can you feel like you can calm your nervous system down so you feel safe? Look at your surroundings. Look at your space or your environment that you are in and try to be in a space that feels safe or calming to you.

Another question you can ask is, is this appropriate? Am I running a marathon right now or am I just doing some very slow restorative strength movements on the floor? Sometimes our brains can make up stories and it's important to remember that you're not running a marathon. You're going to be okay. Particularly if you take a less is more initially approach. If you think you can do a certain amount and be okay with it, halve it again and start there. Meaning do 50% less than what you think you can do. That way you can feel comfortable doing what you're doing, plus the added benefit is you will be more consistent on the daily. Which means more progress long term.

Language is also super important. There's a difference between "I am" versus "I have." *I am fearful of exercise* or *I have a fear of exercise.* The 'I am" statement feels very deep and ingrained, whereas the "I have" lessens it a little. While our brains are very complex, in some ways they are also simple computers. Whatever narrative you tell yourself, your brain will believe. So if you are scared of exercising and then something hurts while you're doing it, your brain validates that fear, strengthens the story you've created, and you might be too scared to continue with the movement. Whereas if you started with the belief that you "have" a fear of exercise, you might still know that movement is going to be good for you and you're doing the appropriate amount. Then when something hurts, you will have no qualms about bringing the intensity down and moving on from that very easily.

Another example is saying, "I am a messy person" versus "I can be messy." Years ago, I was trying to change my behavior and habits around not being messy but had always told myself - *I'm a messy person.* I was trying to change it because I realized if I wanted to be a better leader for my team and expand the program then I better step up and become more organized.

During that time I was at a local cafe talking to one of the baristas. She randomly asked me, "Toby, are you an organized person?"

I said, "Oh no, I'm terribly unorganized." And I caught myself with that language and noticed how bad that was, because I was still associating myself with a trait that I didn't want. I said, "Actually, no, I take that back. I used to be a messy, unorganized person but I'm now becoming more organized."

What was unbelievable was that day I actually started to become more organized. Then the next day I became even more organized, and now I'm super organized. I'm now an organized person. Again, our brains believe anything we tell it, so we can use this to our advantage when trying to change behaviors of deep-seated beliefs. (This is the science behind affirmations and gratitude, by the way.)

Do you know what fear stands for? False Evidence Appearing Real.

Every single success story has stopped focusing on what they can't do and instead used their energy to focus on what they could do. Over time, it compounds everything and with consistency and time, you'll be hiking, bike riding, doing things you have only dreamed of and finally living your life and creating your dream reality.

But it's by focusing on what you can do and nurturing that until you build more capacity.

Movement can look completely different from one person to another. It is completely individualized and it's about understanding that. Understanding what movement is and how we can make it be a positive shift as opposed to the fear factor we often have with chronic fatigue or other health conditions. The one thing I always say is to enjoy movement. We want to have a positive relationship with movement, so enjoy it. Enjoy the process. The process is not linear. Listen to your body.

TAKEAWAYS

STRENGTH IS VITAL TO RECOVERY AND HEALTH: One of the biggest problems with chronic fatigue syndrome is the deconditioning of the body; therefore, reconditioning your body is an integral step of recovery. The more muscle mass you have, the more energy is stored in your body.

FIND YOUR WHY: If we have something driving us to move, we're more likely to do it, we're more likely to enjoy it, and we can see that goal at the end. So before you start your journey, find *why* you want to get strong. For many people, it's because it will be the best way to help them get their life back.

THE DIFFERENT TYPES OF MOVEMENT: The recovery process will most likely start with daily functional movement before moving on to structured movement like cardio and strength training. Just like finding your why, figuring out what type of movement you enjoy and is right for your baseline is essential for success with consistency. All forms of movement have their benefits for your health, but the secret sauce is a combination of strength and cardio.

MOVEMENT SNACKING: This is a great strategy for when you're just starting to regain intentional movement in your day and it involves putting small movements throughout your day, like standing up and down from the couch a few times at different points throughout the day. It all counts and small things create big things!

MOVEMENT THROUGH THE STAGES OF RECOVERY: Choosing movement that is appropriate to your stage of recovery is absolutely essential to consistent growth. In stage 1, we're prioritizing rest and daily functional movement, perhaps with some exercise snacking in there. In stage 2, we can move onto structured movement in small doses, and then stage 3 is when we can do more substantial sessions.

THE RIGHT TYPE OF MUSCULAR FATIGUE: Everyone gets tired and a little sore after structured movement, but it's important for you to recognize when this exceeds the "normal" level and into the painful level where you've overdone it and have more severe CFS symptoms. We don't want you to feel any worse than when you started, and DOMs (delayed onset muscle soreness) should only feel like slight soreness for 1–2 days before subsiding. It shouldn't interfere with your daily function or be so painful you need to wind down your structured movement.

REPLENISH AND RECOVER: There are many ways to recover while doing movement training. You might eat something high in protein (this helps your body to repair those micro tears more efficiently), do magnesium or Epsom salt baths (reduces soreness) or stick your legs up on the wall (helps with blood flow). These are all really good for soothing your muscles after a big session. After doing any form of movement or "energy out" activity, it is recommended to follow it up with something that recharges your battery.

RECOVERY INSPIRATION

Check out this video on the dos and don'ts of exercising with chronic fatigue syndrome.

CHAPTER 10

All Things Progress

One step forward, three steps back. Sound familiar? No it's not the tango or line-dancing, it's the "progress struggle" dance with chronic fatigue syndrome.

Let's face it, having CFS is a challenging circumstance. It's a pretty shit card to be dealt. You can't control the cards you've been dealt but you can still control how you play your hand.

Making progress is different for every single person. It depends on many factors and there's no "one size fits all" for progress.

However, there is a process I call the Pathway to Progress framework, which I will share with you below.

It doesn't matter where you're at, what matters is starting where you are at and what you do with where you're currently at.

As author Stephen Fry once said, "Even if we take three steps forward and two and a half back it's still going half a foot forward."

Forward is forward. And sometimes forward takes us backwards and then forwards, or backwards-backwards and then forward. Progress isn't just a comfortable curve going upwards all the time; often it takes peaks and valleys. Ideally, we want a smoother transition to progress but sometimes these backwards steps are learning lessons so you can move forward with more awareness and insight.

MOVING FORWARD FROM YOUR BASELINE

When it comes to making progress, there's a couple of things we need to think about. One is that it's possible; and the other is that we change our approach from trying to progress *all the time*. We have to include maintenance periods in order for progress to occur.

It's important to adapt to our daily output based on how you feel and the capacity we have on any given day. And this mindset takes practice.

Growing up, sport was my thing. My identity was playing basketball, having a fit body, and being a sporty type of person. Even when I was going through CFS, I was trying to maintain that identity (even if my body was clearly telling me to slow down). My mind had an identity to uphold and I would constantly push my body beyond its limits to try and keep up with my previous fitness and sporting abilities. I refused to relinquish my sporty identity.

If I had a good day, I would push myself way beyond my capacity and then pay for it later (insert major delayed onset muscle soreness and complete crash landings into being bedridden). I got stuck in a vicious cycle where I would rest an entire week and then play a basketball game at 110% only to feel like crap for another week in bed. This push-crash cycle kept me stuck for a very long time, until I became aware of progressive overload and maintenance cycles. Once I figured this out, it unlocked progress like never before. But my point is, progress didn't come without some identity-shattering moments and awareness about what I could or couldn't manage.

If you think about a high-level athlete, they rarely train at 100%. Instead, they're adaptable and restrict their level of output on a weekly basis so they can work every day to gradually build their capacity and fitness. A marathon runner doesn't just get up and run 42.2km at warped speed. If they gave 100% every day, they would be exhausted, unable to recover effectively, and not perform well. They plan their progress. They track their progress, they work towards their progress.

I want you to treat yourself like an athlete who is following a rehabilitation program. If they were coming back from a physical injury, they wouldn't expect to be running at their peak performance, and neither should you. For someone with CFS, the tank is likely already running on empty, so the worst thing you can do is exhaust it more.

As we covered in previous chapters, you need to find your sweet spot, your baseline, and keep it flexible and consistent. What will be most detrimental to your recovery is swinging between full rest and full activity.

THE PATHWAY TO PROGRESS FRAMEWORK

Using the Pathway to Progress framework is a simple way to make progress without derailing your recovery.

Here's what I want you to do. Each time you increase from your baseline, I want you to stop and write down this question.

- ***Does this (increase/next step) feel appropriate for me with where I am right now?***

That's not about where you used to be, or what you were once used to doing…but appropriate for where you are *right now*. Remember you are not comparing your old life to your current capacity.

Firstly you want to avoid the extreme ups and downs.

In order for you to make long lasting progress, you need to stop over-doing it all the time as this will put you in an energy deficit. As Bruce Lee said, "Long-term consistency trumps short-term intensity."

This is a depiction of what NOT to do.

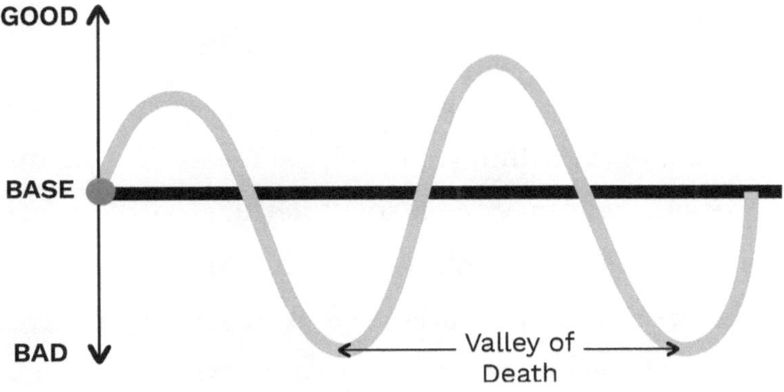

To make progress, you need a foundation to progress from. I see too many people trying to progress before they have a base. So instead of trying to progress right away, you need to make sure you have built a solid baseline that you have been consistent in for at least two to four weeks.

At CFS Health, our Pathway to Progress framework requires members **to maintain their health and current capacity consistently for a minimum of two to four weeks at a time, without feeling any worse than they currently do.**

That timeframe is a marker of safety and stability and it enables you to feel good and see progress while avoiding old tendencies to overdo things and derail progress.

If you do that, progress should look like this:

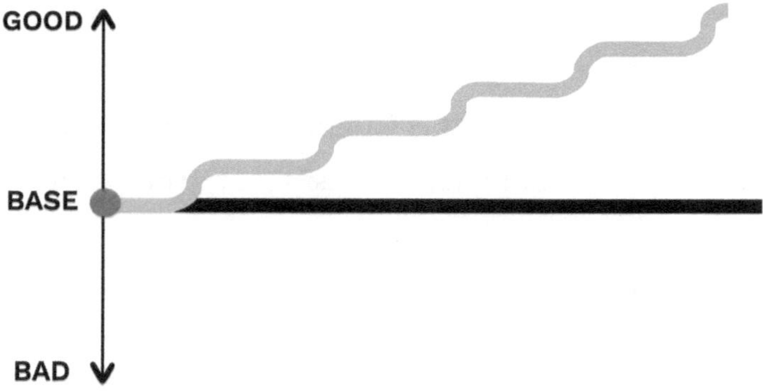

So you can hold and continue to progress, you must include maintenance months within your progress weeks. During maintenance periods, you may see a small flat line on the progress graph each month. This isn't a bad thing, in fact it's a good thing. **Maintenance periods are a sign of progress.** Remember this means maintaining your health and current capacity consistently for a minimum of two to four weeks at a time, without feeling any worse than you currently do. Doing this ensures your brain and body adapts appropriately to your new level of progress. Once it has adapted then you can increase your capacity load appropriately to the new level.

It's important to note that all areas of recovery require energy, whether that be physical, cognitive, mental/emotional or spiritual. So when it comes to progressing, you want to be mindful to not try and progress in all areas at once. Initially, pick one or two areas to work on. Over time, as your capacity expands, you can start to progress in all four key areas more.

Once you increase your load appropriately, you can introduce a maintenance phase of two to four weeks again and continue the process. Rinse and repeat provided that your health is maintained.

It's simple, but simple doesn't mean easy.

How much progress is made varies depending on what stage of recovery you are in.

For instance, if you are in stage 1 of recovery, we recommend not progressing too much as the goal is to stop the push-crash cycle.

The rate in which you progress will continue to change and increase over time.

For people in stage 1 who are at a lower capacity, a good rule is to only progress by 5-20% each time. The good news is the 5-20% rule doesn't apply forever. As you progress through the 3 stages of recovery, your ability to progress faster increases because

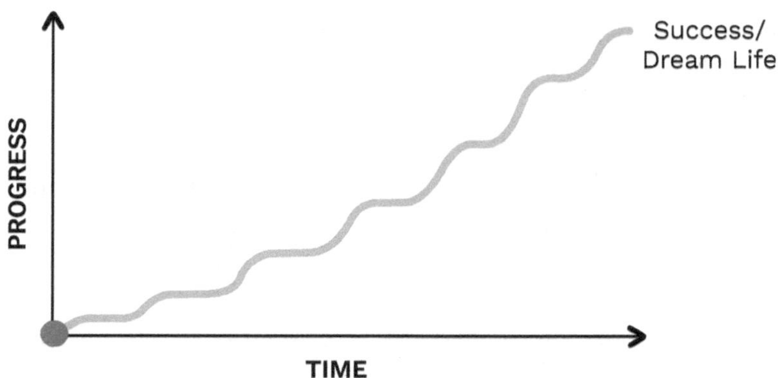

your brain and body gets better at adapting to new stimuli.

As the brain and body become more resilient, it naturally becomes easier and faster to progress as you move from stage 1 to 2, and stage 2 to 3.

It's important not to get fixated on percentages for progress. The 5-20% rule is just a simple framework to ensure you don't overdo it initially. Remember when I said less is more at the beginning?

This is about you being consistent on a daily and weekly basis with your baseline. Over time you will learn the body wisdom to know what to do and when to do it.

As you get better, the 5-20% rule won't be as relevant as you start to make larger progress increments particularly when you move into the lifestyle integration phase. I'll share more about integrating back into life in the next chapter.

As an example, inside our program we have specifically laid out a step by step 12-level restrengthening/reconditioning program that ensures appropriate progression throughout one's recovery. That means our clients aren't second guessing their next progress steps. Initially the progress jumps are smaller but as the levels increase so does your capacity, strength, and stamina. Personalized guidance and specific progress steps are vital for reconditioning as this is not a one-size-fits-all approach and there are many factors at play.

FACTORS THAT CAN INFLUENCE YOUR BASELINE AND PROGRESS

Recovery is not linear and it can be common to have energy dips or crashes during the journey. It's important to take a broad view and not become disheartened. They can happen for a multitude of reasons, but we can actually learn from them by using them as a form of feedback for what is not working for you right now. Other times a setback will be out of your control (like catching the flu or a stressful life event happening), and you will need to learn how to adapt to these appropriately.

**Your baseline is not a rigid rule—
it's a responsive guide.**

Remember how I showed you the RPE scale in chapter 9 (Movement). You want to use the RPE scale every day to tune into your body and scale back certain activities or levels of intensity depending on what's happening in your life and health. As your body and environment shift, so too must your expectations.

**Adjusting your baseline isn't a sign of
failure; it's a sign of wisdom, self-regulation,
and long-term energy preservation.**

Below are five key factors that can commonly impact your baseline. Understanding these can help you stay attuned to your needs, avoid crashes, and help you sustain your current baseline enabling you to progress further over time.

1. Sleep quality

We know that poor sleep reduces your body's ability to restore energy, regulate mood and manage cognitive load, so if you've had several nights of disrupted sleep, you will be functioning at a slightly lower capacity than normal. When this happens, don't force yourself into "normal" activity. Lower your activity expectations. While you definitely don't need to stop everything, it can be helpful to choose more "energy in" activities and reduce the intensity, duration, or number of "energy out" ones. For example, shorten your daily ten-minute walk to five-minutes, or split it into two chunks over the day. This also involves a key mindset shift. Remember that ***rest is productive and flexibility is protective.***

2. Food and nutrition

Skipping meals or eating poorly can lead to energy crashes,

brain fog, and emotional instability, so if you've had a few days of erratic eating or low appetite, recognize this may reduce your capacity. Gently nourish yourself with grounding, easy-to-digest meals that sustain your energy levels and don't leave you feeling like crap afterwards. Remember food is fuel!

3. Stress levels

Your nervous system's stress load changes daily and it impacts everything from energy to digestion to immunity. When your body is under stress (e.g., grief, arguments, big life transitions), it pulls resources away from recovery and toward survival. This makes your energy credits shrink. This can often come from external factors outside of our control, but what we can control is our response to it and our risk minimization strategies. During high-stress periods, cut back your baseline to the essentials. Prioritize rest, "energy in" activities and supportive relationships.

4. Menstrual cycle (if applicable)

Hormonal fluctuations can significantly affect fatigue, mood, and resilience—especially with chronic illness. As we discussed in an earlier chapter, the luteal and menstruation phases of the menstruation cycle can bring increased fatigue, emotional sensitivity and physical pain/discomfort from cramps and bloating. Track your cycle and expect to reduce your baseline during these times (even people without CFS reduce their capacity in these times, switching intense workouts for yoga and increasing their calorie intake). Choose more low-intensity movements, enjoy more "energy in" activities (like journaling, watching light TV, coloring in etc) and increase your calorie intake. Your normal baseline energy days will return—plan for variability, not perfection. Your body is cyclical, not linear. Flow with it, don't fight it.

5. Virus/infections illnesses (cold, flu etc)

Even healthy people slow down when sick—and your system needs even more gentleness during these times. Illnesses like colds or flus place extra demands on an already sensitive system. Continuing your normal baseline during a cold or virus can lead to extended crashes or even relapses. Pull your baseline right back. Focus only on rest, nourishment, and comfort. Let go of all "shoulds." Think…*What would a healthy person do?* They'd rest and look after themselves until they were well again, then they would ease back into life. Do the same for your recovery.

You need to factor these in when it comes to being flexible with your baseline. Tune into your body and use body wisdom to make sure you do what's appropriate. Long-term you'll be thankful you did.

WHAT DOES PROGRESS LOOK LIKE?

Doing new things requires more of your brain and body's energy. It takes time, so please do not be disheartened if you haven't made noticeable progress in the first 4 weeks. It can take a minimum of 8 weeks of consistency for your body to physiologically adapt appropriately and positively in the direction of your goals.

The key indicator of progression is that your health is maintained; meaning that you are not feeling any worse than you currently do. You're not getting sick with colds and flus and your immune system isn't getting compromised. That is a sign that your health is maintaining, and you are fine to continue what you're doing and progress appropriately. On the other hand, getting a cold or flu more than usual can be a sign that you are doing too much or your approach isn't comprehensive enough.

We often look for either huge, mind-blowing progress or none at all. Sometimes we don't even notice our progress and that can be disheartening, so it's important to reflect often on how you're feeling compared to how you used to and appreciate how far you've come.

Identifying signs of progress is a positive ritual you can do to feel nourished through the process. I have made a list of 277 signs of progress that I will share with you in the Recovery Inspiration section at the end of this chapter (yes, no progress goes undetected…here are a few noticeable ones to get you started.

Some common signs of progress include:
- your symptoms are less intense or persistent
- your sleep is better
- your mental capacity is better than six months ago
- you're laughing more and your personality is returning
- you're less reactive
- your poo is better—yes, healthy poos means progress!
- you're more engaged in daily life

We are often the last ones to notice progress within ourselves and it's important to remember that progress doesn't always have to be physical. It can be cognitive, social, emotional, spiritual and hormonal. It can be super helpful to keep a diary on how you're feeling day in and day out (try to avoid listing symptoms and instead focus on how you *feel*. For example, *I felt a small burst of energy after breakfast this morning. I did the dishes and felt okay afterwards, and I really enjoyed my ten-minute walk. I did hit a low at around 3 p.m. and had a thirty-minute sleep but I woke up feeling marginally better.* This will help you identify ways that your life has improved, say if you look back three or four months on and you're now walking twenty minutes and you forgot that you had started at ten. Make sure to acknowledge any and all wins you have and celebrate them.

When it comes to progress there are four key areas of progress. Here are some examples within each category so you can see if you are on the right track.

Physical Progress:
- more functional around the house
- doing more and feeling no worse for it
- increased capacity for socializing
- increase in strength and stamina
- increased capacity for daily chores
- needing less sleep during the day
- waking up earlier

- sitting up more
- standing more
- cooking more meals
- increase in libido
- doing tasks for longer
- working again
- increase in work hours
- studying again
- improved menstrual and hormonal balance
- healthier digestive system
- more capacity for restorative strength training
- increased ability to stretch
- walking
- biking
- increase in body strength
- participation in training or sport

Cognitive progress

- reading a book for longer
- watching TV for longer
- listening to a podcast for longer
- conversing and socializing
- studying or focusing
- learning something new
- playing an instrument
- starting a new career

- returning to work
- playing board games such as chess or Scrabble
- getting better at memory retention through games and learning
- increased screentime with ease
- increased capacity for learning

Mental/Emotional progress
- better emotional regulation in hard situations
- a more optimistic outlook on life
- more balanced emotions
- doing less cognitive distortions (for example: catastrophizing—expecting the worst; overgeneralizing—using an isolated negative event to draw a broad, negative conclusion; and black-and-white thinking—seeing things as only good or bad.
- better at setting boundaries
- decrease in guilt and shame
- more relaxation in the nervous system
- better emotional responses versus knee-jerk reactions
- reacting less, responding more
- looking towards the future more
- focusing on building a new life instead of wishing for the old one
- increased self-awareness
- less people-pleasing and more personal empowerment

Spiritual/Inner self progress
- experiencing a deeper sense of self
- a deeper connection to your personal values
- an increased sense of meaning
- more perspective on what's truly important to you
- being pulled towards the life you want versus forcing it
- a deeper relationship with God, faith, universe, religion
- more aligned friendships and relationships
- deeper conversations that matter to you
- more listening to the innate wisdom your body and mind are telling you
- feeling more purpose and passion

Small steps toward progress are recommended, especially when you're starting out. Just like if you had an injury, the same goes for outperforming your capacity: you wouldn't expect to run a marathon tomorrow if the furthest you've ever run is 5 kilometers, would you? I find a lot of people jump the gun. They go super fast too quickly and then they pay for it and feel horrible. But there's another way, and the other way is to do it appropriately.

Start with the minimum effective dose initially and then build from there. This means that you start at the bare minimum of what feels simple and appropriate for you. Remember less is more initially and being consistent is going to be the fastest way for you to get better. If you keep going beyond your baseline and current capacity too quickly, you're shooting yourself in the foot. Stop red-lining and get on the green line with your baseline!

I always suggest to my clients to do half as much as they think they can do. That's usually a good starting point.

We often overestimate what we can do in a short period of time, but under-estimate what we can do over a long period of time.

Here are some examples of what it could look like day-to-day:

Day to day cognitive progress

Let's imagine you first started reading again, and you could get to four pages before your brain started slowing down and getting tired. This would leave you feeling foggy for a while afterwards. So instead, just read one page. Do this for a week or two and see how you feel. One day, you'll notice that you feel good after reading that one page. You will naturally feel a pull to read a little more once you have maintained that for two to four weeks. After that, you can progress your reading by either time or pages depending on how you want to track progress. You might read an extra half of a page in your next progress period, then you would maintain that for two to four weeks (making sure the key five factors aren't getting in the way of your recovery and you can keep progressing from there).

A client named Haily from the UK couldn't even look at a book because she was so sick with CFS when she started our program. We helped her find her baseline. One of her main goals was to enjoy reading again. She started with reading just a couple of sentences a day. As the weeks progressed, so did her baseline and cognitive capacity. She increased her reading over time. She progressed so much within two years that she went from not being able to look at a book to reading an entire book within three weeks! And the book was huge!

Little by little can become a lot. When you do the right things at the right time, you get the right results.

And don't forget that each time you increase your capacity, you want to ask yourself, **is this *doable, appropriate and maintainable* (D.A.M)?**

Day to day sleep progress

Progress doesn't have to be thought of in terms of addition either, as it can also be about decreasing certain activities, like how much you sleep, particularly during the day. Let's say you're sleeping during the day and you want to work toward not having day-time naps. The first step to this would be decreasing your sleep by 10 to 15 minutes for your day time nap and maintaining that level of decreased day-time sleep for one to two weeks, adjusting accordingly to what feels right. You will then keep bringing it down slightly by that ten to fifteen minutes until you reach your goal. You could also swap your daytime sleeps for more rest periods throughout the day, and as you start to get even better, those rest periods will become less frequent. All good signs of progress. Then do a little check-in, and ask yourself: **is this *doable, appropriate and maintainable for me?* Consistency is the key!**

Day to day emotional progress

You might also need to pull back from a relationship you find stressful. Maybe it's a family member or friend who comes to visit and rants for two hours while they are there, leaving you emotionally drained. You could start by setting boundaries with either time or content. For instance, asking them to only stay for an hour or telling them that you'd like to only discuss positive things when they visit. Having boundaries for your capacity is an act of self-love and self-care. Emotional drainers can wreak havoc with your equilibrium, so consider ways you can reduce stressful relationship issues and extend self-care.

Remember to always check in and ask yourself: **is this *doable, appropriate and maintainable for me?***

Day to day physical progress

For physical progress, it may be slightly progressing your restorative strength training program from a few minutes in bed to five minutes on a yoga mat. Once you're there, continually increase the time by small increments (only a couple of minutes) and monitor how you feel after each session to make sure that was the appropriate amount.

As mentioned in Chapter 9, Movement using the RPE framework for physical movement and activities enables safe progression over time. Whether that be gardening, gym, dancing, rock climbing, hiking, biking. You name it; it's doable.

You may start off with a gentle walk and an exertion of three or four out of ten in terms of energy output. You maintain that for two to four weeks and then you may be able to walk for a little bit longer or increase to a four or five exertion level of out ten.

As you get stronger and your capacity starts to increase, you can choose a specific area of progress and build on it.

Remember again to check in and ask yourself: **is this *doable, appropriate and maintainable for me?***

ALEX

I had a client called Alex who is now a mentor at CFS Health. When she was first in her recovery phase, she would say, "Toby, I *really* want to run. I'm walking for ten minutes, and now I'm going to run for ten minutes."

I knew this wasn't a great idea. I said, "Alex. I know you love running but I suggest you do your ten-minute walk first, and build that up. Maybe slowly add another minute or two of walking and see how that feels first. Make sure your health is maintained for two more weeks and build up to the comfortability of around fifteen to twenty minutes of walking. Is that appropriate and doable?"

"Yes!" she replied, she was on board.

Once Alex hit twenty minutes of walking and *it felt good*, I said, "What I want you to do is now sneak in a few moments of light jogs within your walk, to the point where you're not forcing anything but feeling the sensation of what it feels like to do a light jog within your walk. To start with just a few strides or maybe it's ten steps of jogging, and then you go back to your normal walk, and then you'll do maybe another few strides or ten seconds of jogging five minutes later and you'll continue on in that pattern. Come back to me in a couple of weeks and let's see how you're going."

Alex beamed. She was excited to try a few light jogging steps. After 2 weeks, Alex sent me a message saying, *Toby, I did it. And It actually felt really good to run without feeling exhausted or burnt out.*

These micro changes paid off and Alex was jogging on and off for five kilometers within five months. Consistency over intensity is the key!

It's all about giving the brain and the body appropriate stimulus for it to adapt well.

If you try to make outrageous changes that are too big, the brain and body can't handle that amount of load initially and instead of responding well, they'll react and cause a flare up in symptoms.

This is how the brain and body tries to protect itself from threats. We have to create safety in the brain and the body for them to respond appropriately. Alex took the advice well and as a result her brain and body responded well.

Little by little, becomes a lot.

Key tip: You are not starting over every time you lower your baseline. You are working with your body, not against it. When you respect your limits, your limits tend to expand gently over time provided you do the right things at the right time. When you ignore them, they shrink.

Your baseline isn't about doing more—it's about doing what's right for you right now.

SETBACK STRATEGIES

Below are some strategies you can implement when you need to reduce your baseline as a result of a crash or setback:

1. **Relax and go back to basics:** Setbacks can feel overwhelming, but the key is to *not panic*. It's easy to get caught up in over-analyzing everything when you're not feeling your best. But the first step is to simply go back to basics. Don't overcomplicate things. Start by focusing on the simple, foundational steps you already know help you. Sometimes your body needs rest, and that's okay. Remember, your body is asking for a break—it's not a failure.

2. **Rest, relax, and do a little:** It's easy to slip into an "all-or-nothing" mindset with CFS, but that's not helpful. You don't have to do everything, but you also don't have to do nothing. Find balance. If you're feeling low, do what you can. Even if it's getting a glass of water or sitting outside for 10 minutes, that's progress. Stop searching online for more problems, and instead, give yourself permission to rest and do small, manageable things. Cognitive overload is a real thing, and we want to make sure you're giving your brain and body the rest it needs. Stop doctor-googling every symptom and every problem. If you are in a setback your brain and body is asking for calmness and relaxation. Cognitive overload is a real thing where you're constantly bombarding your brain with information. So much so you don't even retain any of it but just stress yourself out even more.

3. **Fuel your body with the right food:** Food is fuel for your body, especially when dealing with CFS. When you're in a setback, focus on eating foods you know work for you. If you've tracked your energy levels and symptoms with different foods, go back to what gives you consistent energy and avoid what doesn't. Mealtimes and frequency matter, too. You might need to eat every two to three hours to maintain and fuel your brain and body with more sustained energy levels. Listen to your body and give it what it needs without stressing about it. Remember food is fuel after all.

4. **Sleep and rest smart:** Sleep is crucial, but it's about finding the right balance. If you need to sleep during the day, go for it, but try to sleep between 11am and 3pm so it doesn't interfere with your nighttime sleep. Over time, as you heal, you may find that you need less daytime sleep and can rely more on night sleep. But for now, listen to your body and give it the rest it's asking for.

5. **Use positive language:** The words you say to yourself and others have a huge impact on your mindset and recovery. If you find yourself saying, "I don't know if this will ever end," stop, and flip it. Instead, say, "I'm healing," or "I just need to look after myself, and I'll bounce back." The narrative you create around your illness matters. Avoid getting stuck in a negative mindset and shift to a more supportive, positive one. Don't let a bad morning ruin a good day, don't let a bad day ruin a good week, don't let a bad week ruin a good month.

6. **Relaxation practices:** In CFS recovery, relaxation is key. One simple technique is legs up the wall—a gentle stretch where you lie down with your legs against the wall. This helps blood flow, especially back to your brain, and switches on the parasympathetic nervous system (the rest and digest state). Even five minutes of this can help you feel more relaxed and grounded. Pair it with deep breathing or meditation if that feels good

for you too. You can try other calming methods like restorative breathing, visualizations, yoga nidra etc.

7. **Hydration and avoiding stimulants:** With CFS, staying hydrated is really important. Sip water throughout the day rather than chugging large amounts all at once. Try to avoid stimulants like caffeine or energy drinks, as they can lead to crashes later on. Instead, opt for calming, non-caffeinated drinks like herbal teas (chamomile, peppermint, etc.) that support your body's relaxation and healing.

8. **Gentle movement:** Even when you're in a setback, a little bit of movement can be helpful, provided it's appropriate for you. It might be a lot less than you normally do in your typical day-to-day baseline. It doesn't have to be much—maybe a stretch on your yoga mat, a short walk outside or a simple play with your dog in your backyard or even just moving from the bed to the couch eventually can be super helpful. Remember, energy eventually creates energy, but you don't want to push too hard. Do what feels right for your body, even if it's a few minutes of light stretching.

9. **Build back slowly:** As you start feeling a bit better, ease back into activity slowly. There's no rush, and you don't need to overanalyze the timing. Listen to your body and

build up at a pace that feels right for you. One of the biggest mistakes people make is setting timelines like, "I'll be back to normal in two weeks." Instead, drop the expectations and focus on small, consistent steps forward. You will be surprised how well you do if you use body wisdom as your guide to return to expanding your capacity. Go gently with compassion and you will bounce back faster.

10. **Journaling and tracking progress:** Keep using your daily planner or journal. It's not about journaling every single day but reflecting when you feel up to it. This helps you stay connected to what works for you and gives you a sense of progress, even in the small things.

Setbacks are a normal part of recovery. It's not about avoiding them, but how you respond to them. Follow these steps, trust your body, and you'll bounce back stronger. Take your time, be kind to yourself, and know that you're making progress even when it feels slow.

THE PROGRESS GAP

Embracing Boredom as a Catalyst for Growth

When you're on the journey of CFS recovery, there comes a time when you hit a plateau—a stage where your baseline is solid, symptoms have eased, and your routine feels predictable. But along with this progress comes an unexpected guest: boredom. Not the kind of boredom that stems from passively binge-watching TV all day, but a deeper restlessness—a sense that you're stuck between where you were and where you want to be.

The fact that you have time to be bored now is a sign of progress. You were once so ill, and consumed by symptoms you didn't have a moment to be bored.

If you find yourself in this "progress gap," or what we like to call the "boredom gap." It is that middle stage of recovery, sandwiched between building your baseline and fully integrating back into life. And here's the surprising truth: **boredom is a sign of progress.** Let's explore why and how you can use it to propel yourself forward.

Why Boredom Is a Good Thing

When you were at your lowest point, boredom wasn't even an option. You were consumed by symptoms, discomfort, and the emotional weight of your illness. The very fact that you can now experience boredom is evidence of progress. It means your symptoms no longer dominate your every waking moment, and you've progressed enough to not be in a state of suffering 24/7. This is a luxury many people in recovery don't recognize as a milestone—but it is.

The Boredom Gap: A Place of Opportunity

The boredom gap is the space between maintenance and momentum. It's where many people feel like they're not progressing, but in reality, they're laying the groundwork for the next phase of recovery. The temptation here is to either settle for "good enough" or to lose patience and push too hard. But what's needed is consistency—doing more of what works, more repetitions and then slowly but progressively doing them at a slightly higher level.

Think of your recovery as climbing a mountain. You've ascended past the difficult base and reached a plateau. The peak, where lifestyle integration awaits, is still ahead. To move forward, you don't need drastic changes: you need steady, intentional effort. Energy creates energy, and small, consistent actions will build momentum.

How to navigate the progress gap

1. **Keep doing what works:** If your current routine has brought you this far, don't abandon it. Instead, refine it. Add small, manageable challenges to stretch yourself gently.

2. **Infuse joy:** Recovery doesn't have to feel like *Groundhog Day*. Find activities that spark joy and replenish energy—playing an instrument, painting, writing, or connecting with friends. Infusing creativity into your day prevents stagnation and makes the process more enjoyable.

3. **Focus on the long game:** Don't measure progress by days or weeks. Instead, show up consistently. Over time, those small efforts compound, leading to big changes. Ignore time. Just keep showing up.

4. **Expand your vision:** We run out of energy when
   we run out of vision. Use this phase to explore what's
   next. What do you want to reintegrate into your life?
   Relationships, work, hobbies, and passions—these are
   the threads of a full life waiting to be woven back in.

5. **Create goals bigger than your current
   circumstance:** "Are you thinking big enough?" This is
   a question I ask my clients who find themselves plateaued
   in the boredom gap. Often they stay "comfortable and
   stuck" vs asking bigger and better questions to expand
   their lives and progress beyond their current reality. Are
   you thinking big enough?

6. **Make sure fear isn't in the way:** people often
   stay stuck in this middle ground of recovery, because
   on the other side of getting better is the fear of being
   fully recovered, fear of having to deal with life and
   responsibilities, or the fear of over-doing it so you stay
   stuck with where you're at. Remember fear stands for
   false evidence appearing real.

Progress Over Perfection

The boredom gap is a normal and necessary stage of recovery.
It's not a sign that you're stuck but that you're ready for more.
Embrace this period as an opportunity to solidify your founda-
tion and gently expand your horizons. Celebrate how far you've

come, but don't settle. Keep choosing progress over perfection, and trust that your steady efforts will lead you to full lifestyle integration.

As you move forward, remember: **boredom isn't the end of the road; it's a doorway to your next level of growth.**

Stay consistent, stay curious, and stay committed. Your best life is waiting just beyond this gap.

TAKEAWAYS

KEY TO MOVING FORWARD: When it comes to making progress, it's important to maintain flexibility and ditch the idea that you can do it all while in recovery. It's important to adapt to your daily output based on how you feel.

INCREASING YOUR BASELINE: Each time you increase from your baseline, I want you to stop and write down this question: *Does this feel appropriate for me with where I am right now?* Really think about it and take note of what your previous output was and make sure you're not increasing too steeply.

MAINTAIN BEFORE YOU PROGRESS: It's important to maintain your new level for a minimum of two to four weeks before you progress again. Remember the brain and body love stability and consistency. Do this and you will progress faster long-term.

PROGRESS TO PATHWAY FRAMEWORK: Remember to not progress too quickly or by too much initially. Use the 5-20% progress guideline to ensure you don't overdo it initially. Knowing that over time as your capacity, strength and stamina increases, the rate in which you progress will too.

FACTORS THAT INFLUENCE YOUR BASELINE: Recovery is not always linear and sometimes setbacks and relapses can be part of the journey. This could be sleep quality, nutrition intake, stress levels, menstrual cycle, minor illnesses. Your baseline is not a rigid rule—it's a responsive guide. It's important to take a broad view and not become disheartened.

YOU ARE NOT STARTING OVER EVERY TIME YOU LOWER YOUR BASELINE: You are working with your body, not against it. When you respect your limits, your limits tend to expand gently over time. When you ignore them, they shrink.

SIGNS YOU ARE MAKING PROGRESS: If you want to make sure that you're progressing, the key indicator here is that your health is maintaining, meaning that you are not feeling any worse than you currently do. Other signs of progress include sleeping better than you used to, dealing with bad days better, increased mental capacity, you have the energy to be bored, and you are less reactive or irritable than you used to be.

EMBRACE BOREDOM: When you're on the journey of CFS recovery, there comes a time when you hit a plateau—a stage where your baseline is solid, symptoms have eased, and your routine feels predictable. But along with this progress comes an unexpected guest: boredom. While it doesn't feel like it, boredom is a sign of progress. When you were at your lowest point, boredom wasn't even an option as you were consumed by symptoms, discomfort, and the emotional weight of your illness. You can navigate this part in your recovery by continuing to do what works, infuse more joy into your daily routine, focus on the long game and expand your vision.

RECOVERY INSPIRATION

Download our free checklist that has 277 tangible signs of progress that your doctor won't be able to tell you.

CHAPTER 11

Lifestyle Integration

There comes a point when you will be ready to begin integrating into "normal" life again. Many people get to this place having previously believed that they never would. And that might be you too, wondering if you'll ever get back living again.

I want to let you know that it's absolutely possible, I see it every single day.

Over the last sixteen years, I have witnessed so many people from all walks of life believing it wasn't possible for them to get better, only to see those same people years later living their lives fully again.

Lifestyle integration marks a turning point in your recovery. What starts to happen as you get better is that you progress to the point of being able to think about life beyond recovery. Things like work or career building, studying, going back to school, socializing, relationships, hobbies, fitness, or travel, start to become your focus. The shift moves from recovery to life. This can be an exciting time and scary time.

On one hand you're excited because you're feeling better, but on the other hand new fears can pop up. Fear of the future, fear that you will do too much and go backwards, fear that you won't know how to live a normal life again.

Getting back to normal life brings its own challenges: paying bills, new responsibilities, navigating old and new relationships, work, study, duties.

NEW LEVEL, NEW DEVIL

Even when life starts to open up, it can feel challenging. Each new level you rise to seems to come with a new challenge. This is perfectly okay and a normal part of life.

So how do you know if you're ready to focus on integrating back into life again? Here are some key indicators:

- You have progressed in your overall capacity. You're no longer focusing on day-to-day recovery because you've progressed beyond surviving each day.
- You've got the basics covered and you've noticed significant progress in your daily capacity which extends beyond the home.
- You're ready to think and explore life beyond your day-to-day basics because you have the energy to do so.
- You're confident in your plan and you feel ready to expand your life beyond recovery.

- Symptoms no longer dictate your days.
- Your current challenges are no longer primarily health related.

For many of our members integrating back into life can take anywhere between six to twelve months. Some take longer, and some shorter. However timeframes aren't the goal and measuring time against recovery puts too much unnecessary pressure on yourself which doesn't help you feel empowered about your journey.

Just stay focused on the process, and the results will come. Don't focus on time.

As one of our recovered members, Andrew said during his success interview—"Drop the clock—stop measuring time against recovery."

Brilliant advice from a man who could barely get out of bed to now fully living again. He's right. You don't need any more pressure than you already have. Having CFS is enough pressure as it is. Drop the clock.

You can watch his full interview here:

As your capacity expands, so does your life. The same principles apply when it comes to progressing further into your new life— make sure you increase things appropriately. The good news is, in stage 3 you will have mastered body wisdom, and for the most part during this stage, energy creates more energy. The bigger your capacity, the faster your progress grows.

NEW LIFE, NEW YOU

Creating your new life means you're not going back to your old one. Part of developing a new life is creating a new vision for yourself. What was important to you before you got sick is most likely not going to be as important as you get better. You may have radically changed your perspective on life. Your values may have shifted and it's good to be clear on what those values are. The experience of chronic illness changes who you are as a person. Often it adds more depth to your experience of life and a newfound gratitude for your health. This is one of the gifts we get from it.

In my 16 years of experience helping people overcome CFS, 99% of people usually change aspects of their life that are completely different from their pre-CFS days. Some people change their career, for others it may be their hobbies or friendship circles. Whatever it is—they have changed into what I call their new 2.0 version. This is an upgraded version of who you are *now* based on the new life you are building and want to live. You're still the same person as you used to be, but just an upgraded, more evolved version. It's like most people find a new way of life that resonates more deeply with who they are now, not who they used to be.

You know what's crazy? I have not met one person who recovered from CFS who wasn't thankful for the experience. It gave them blessings and gifts they once otherwise would not have received. Of course they weren't thrilled about getting CFS, they wouldn't wish it upon their worst enemy, but there was a silver lining and message in the mess that gave them gifts for the rest of their life.

**"Time to open up a new chapter in life,
and to explore a larger center."
—Lillian Russell**

EVOLUTION OF RELATIONSHIPS

Yes, even relationships change. After being unwell for a prolonged period, the dynamics of some of your relationships are likely to have changed. This is particularly true of your intimate relationships or family ones, because the unwell person may have had a certain level of reliance on their loved ones. They became their carers and the support system. As that person starts to get better, their loved ones need to stop checking in on them all the time. (I go into more detail about this in the chapter 12, CFS and Loved Ones).

What happens is that the relationship evolves from dependent to codependent, and the recovered sufferer has gone from "I need you to help me get through the day" to "You're a human being who I love and want in my life, and we're going to do life together."

The opposite can happen too, where you will outgrow certain friendships or relationships that no longer serve you. Particularly if these people are not interested in growing and evolving with you. They may only see and only appreciate the old version of you. And now that you're different and have evolved, they may feel insecure or indifferent to you. None of this is bad or wrong, it's just life.

These are some of the challenges and joys of integrating back into life that no one talks about.

This evolution is a huge journey. There's also a new element of transparent authenticity as you stand up for yourself and what you believe is right for you and what you need in life. It can alter the dynamics of relationships but it can also enhance the relationship you have with yourself. That part is kind of cool.

One client, Timothy, discovered that the main relationship that changed for him was the one he had with himself. When he got sick he was very hard on himself. He was always telling himself of the type of person he used to be. He was fun and outgoing and sporty. Spending time by himself was something he felt uncomfortable with at first. He knew himself as the center of attention, not the introvert he had become. His identity was smashed. He fell into a depression and hated his new life - trapped in his bedroom and isolated and alone. He thought that life was unfair and that he might as well be the victim he was. One of the few things he enjoyed was listening to music. It helped him feel calm and escape his negative thoughts.

One day, he picked up his old guitar that he hadn't touched in years and decided to strum it. He wasn't a guitarist at all. In fact, he gave up trying to play it because sport was more fun.

Slowly and surely, Timothy started to learn a few chords. He had time to learn and no pressure to be good. Some days he played and other days he didn't. But learning the guitar in teeny tiny incremental steps took his mind off things for a short time. It strengthened his fingers and hands and posture and gave him something to look forward to.

Although it took quite some time, Timothy is now recovered. He is also able to play guitar. He believes that he never would have had the patience to learn under "normal circumstances"— but CFS is never considered normal circumstances. It changed him. It changed the relationship Tim had with himself, and with his illness. It gave him a gift in the long run. One he built from the depths of despair in his old life but could integrate into his new life in new and positive ways.

REVISITING YOUR VALUES AND VISION

While you are sick, your focus is on achieving a full recovery. As lifestyle integration begins, it is time to start thinking beyond yourself. In fact, part of the healing journey is not focusing on you all the time. Eventually, the focus will be less inward on yourself and more outward to the world and the people around you.

I often say to members inside our Lifestyle Integration program that part of the recovery journey and integrating back into life is about taking the focus off themselves and onto others. Helping other people when you're in this stage of recovery is actually part of the healing process.

Looking beyond yourself and to the broader world is an incredible experience. It's an adventure. One of the hardest parts of this new adventure is the overwhelm that often comes with it.

Over time, people who are chronically ill start to separate themselves from normal life and their current health becomes the main obstacle. They think how nice it must be to have a family, a job, friends and hobbies, meanwhile, they're not seeing the challenges that come along with a "normal" life, like breakups, financial problems, job insecurity, grief and other life struggles. It can be overwhelming for you as you reintegrate to remember that normal life isn't all roses either.

Life has its fair share of trials and tribulations, and when you integrate back into life, you're no longer sheltered or protected from life's many challenges.

We receive letters and gifts in the mail all the time from our members all around the world. Recently a card landed on my desk from one of our lovely members named Brendan.

On the card it had a drawing of a rainbow. Inside the card there were some words from Brendan. It said the following:

Like the miraculous appearance of a beautiful rainbow, beneath the last of the dark and grumbling storm clouds…We emerge from the depths of the CFS curse to become someone and create a life even more wonderful than we could imagine.

He went on to give his thanks to my team, the program, and to me for the work we do at CFS health.

A little rainbow to help celebrate the global ecosystem of healing, discovery, and self fulfillment you have created together.

Powerful words.

It got me thinking, *Brendan is right. You can't have a rainbow without the storm clouds.*

And even getting your life back comes with storm clouds.

Part of decreasing the overwhelm and handling the storm clouds is going back to your values, and remembering what is important to you, and prioritizing it.

One of the big struggles many people face when they start to integrate back into life, is they can do many more things and they want to play "catch up." So they want to do everything! Because let's face it…they've been dreaming of all the things they want to do for so long. But remember—even healthy people can't do everything they want to do all the time. You have to stay very intentional and clear on what you *really* want to do and what matters versus what isn't a high priority right now.

The other key is to keep doing the things that help you feel good. So many people fall backwards because they stop doing the things that help them feel good in the first place.

Remember, health is a forever thing, recovery doesn't have to be. Just because you're better or getting better, doesn't mean you stop focusing on your health and wellbeing.

My mantra for avoiding overwhelm is "prioritize, delegate or delay." There is a tendency for people to make up for lost time and they can start to do too much. There is travel to do, marathons to run, bucket list items to tick, and people to see. It is important *not* to do everything at once. Choose what matters to you right now and build on that.

Something else that helps with mindset during the process of reintegration is recognizing that there are two types of challenges in the world. There are challenges chosen for us and challenges we get to choose. The first type is something like chronic fatigue syndrome. It's not what you wanted. You didn't choose it. It just happened. It sucks, but you have to deal with it.

What I call a "choice challenge" is something you're purposefully working towards and is usually a fun goal or a goal you want to achieve for the sake of your interest and values, like a desire to become an awesome piano player or learn a new language or to get stronger so you can hike mountains or play sport. The great thing is that you get to choose where to invest your energy. You can exercise your choice muscle and decide what gets your energy and what does not.

ANNE

One of our members Anne is an incredible example of exercising choice and vision. Anne says, "prior to being unwell I was incredibly fit and active, when not working internationally, I was competing in Ironman events."

But when Anne suddenly became unwell her whole life changed. Her speech was impaired, she couldn't lift her head or even use a pillow, she had severe light sensitivity and constantly wore an eye mask. Her partner had to give up work to look after her.

When she joined our membership program she described herself as "one of those members with a one-sided face. The ones you see online in the sessions laying flat on the bed resting on one side of their face staring at the screen or falling asleep."

Recovery took time, but Anne took the journey. Step by little step. It was a full integration process.

One time, during our program one of our coaches suggested that Anne write about her "future life—what life would look like for her fully recovered. Anne took on that challenge and wrote pages and pages of detail.

She recalls me asking her to "invest in things that will help you arrive at your vision." (This was later on in the process when it was appropriate to suggest this to Anne).

Fast-forward to 2025 and Anne sent me an update on her life. She is unstoppable. She recently trekked for 26 days and delighted in every moment. She said it was "tougher than expected, perilous in sections, glorious, memorable, exhausting, invigorating and funny." But the amazing thing is that while trekking Anne realized that her life was exactly as she had written in detail as her "dream life" when she could hardly speak or lift her head. Isn't that powerful?!

She is now planning for her physical challenge and adventure.

She sent me a text that said: *I am forever grateful for the period I spent with you all. Not only have I physically recovered but the new version of me is someone I love spending time with. I live in the moment, I am grateful for everything life offers, I am so much kinder to myself, I live within my boundaries, I invest my time and resources into what matters to me versus what I once thought I was expected to do.*

FINDING PURPOSE

Life after illness often comes with a renewed sense of perspective. For me, recovery meant I couldn't simply be content with having a job and earning money. The devastation that came with CFS changed me forever. I never wanted anyone else to suffer the way I did. Starting CFS Health was purpose-driven from the very start. It was a calling that extended beyond me and my illness. It gave me a deeper sense of purpose and a bigger reason for living through those tumultuous years.

Many of my clients are now CFS Health mentors, in fact 95% of our coaches had CFS, went through our program, recovered, and now work for CFS Health giving back and helping others. Not because they need a job but because having CFS changed them forever and now they want to help others have a good quality of life that they are now experiencing.

See, your journey with CFS was purposeful, reframe your experience so it can serve to help rather than hinder. Maybe it has made you a more compassionate person, a kinder person, a gentler and more patient person. Seeing purpose in the pain is a transformative shift. It certainly changed the course of my life, and I believe having a purpose or creating one will be one of the most enriching experiences of your life if you allow it.

CARVE OUT BOUNDARIES

An important part of integrating into life is finding inner certainty. As you recover, you become more self-led and what I call the "true you." You are free to make your own choices, whereas when you are sick you often have to delegate choices to your body (how you were feeling that day decided what you were able to do). It's short-term pain for long-term gain.

But with choices comes great responsibility! Many people find it necessary to carve out their boundaries and re-establish their new values of what matters to them; doing this enables them to focus on creating a life they love. Saying no to things that your sick self would have jumped at the opportunity to do takes a lot of work and practice, but it's important to only do things that you *want* to do or need to do, not what you think you *should* do now that you're better. It is important to keep at it because boundaries are intertwined with being true to yourself and ultimately maintaining good health.

Carving out boundaries and learning to say no, without any kind of over-explanation or apology, is a really important step for many people in their healing journey. The ability to say no is actually health promoting and beneficial for your well-being, even after your initial recovery stages. It is also often an issue for parents as they put their family's needs ahead of their own every single time, but it can be beneficial and empowering for both parent and child to explain why they need to prioritize themselves at that point.

**If you can't put yourself first,
at least put yourself equal.**

Guilt is a heavy emotion, probably one of the heaviest we experience. Imagine having a backpack filled with rocks that is weighing you down. It doesn't matter how healthy you are, how nice you are, if your sleep is perfect and if you're doing everything right, you're still walking around with a heavy backpack of what I call guilt rocks. You're not going to move forward until you ditch the guilt rocks.

If you want some inspiration from people just like you, I interviewed three incredible humans who re-integrated back into life and they share their best tips here:

**Creating your new life means embracing the
new version of yourself and building the new.
Let go of the old and create a new reality that
you could only dream of. Recovery is possible.**

TAKEAWAYS

REINTEGRATING INTO "NORMAL" LIFE IS A CRUCIAL TURNING POINT IN RECOVERY: Once you're starting to feel better and have progressed in your overall capacity, it's time to shift from constantly prioritizing recovery to integrating into the world around you.

AS YOU HEAL, RELATIONSHIPS EVOLVE: This is especially true with loved ones, as you shift from a dependence-based dynamic to a more equal partnership. During this process, it's also essential to revisit your values and vision for life, which may have shifted after your experience with illness. Often, this results in finding more meaningful work or new passions and learning to set boundaries as you navigate reintegration.

REINTEGRATION CAN FEEL OVERWHELMING: You can get bogged down with comparison, but by focusing on your core values and prioritizing what matters most, you can manage the overwhelm. Learning to carve out boundaries, say no without guilt, and embrace your true self helps you create a balanced life, free from the pressures of trying to be everything to everyone.

MOVE TOWARDS MORE OF WHAT YOU WANT: It's about no longer wishing for your old life back, but rather building a new life that is aligned with who you are now, your current values and goals that matter to you now.

RECOVERY INSPIRATION

Scan here to watch a bunch of success stories, people from all walks of life who have integrated back into life.

CHAPTER 12

CFS and Loved Ones

It is often as hard for a loved one to see you suffer as it is for you to go through it. I remember how upset my mom was. She often said, "Toby, I wish I could change bodies with you." She meant it too.

I'm one of the lucky ones, my parents were, and still are, super supportive. That's not everyone's experience. Many of my clients have shared how their family members found it hard to fully understand their illness. It can cause a lot of tension when there's a lack of understanding, knowledge, and support around CFS.

I've written this chapter to address some of this lack of understanding. It can be handy to bookmark and pass it to a family member to read. It may help them understand the "invisible illness" that you are currently experiencing.

UNDERSTANDING THE COMPLEXITY OF CHRONIC FATIGUE SYNDROME

What happens with chronic fatigue syndrome is that you're living a normal life when a bunch of things happen! It could be work, stress, a virus infection, a traumatic event or several traumatic events over a period of time. Things start spiraling downhill. Usually it's either one thing or a bunch of things that happen over a period of time and suddenly the brain and body can't handle the load anymore.

As a result, your immune system gets worse and eventually your brain and body goes into shutdown mode. It's bewildering and shocking. You get a bunch of symptoms—usually eight or more, that persist for a period of six months before you get diagnosed. And what happens is that you're not only dealing with the symptoms, but you're also dealing with a hurricane of emotional chaos.

Chronic fatigue syndrome isn't in the mind. It's a real neurological and physical illness. People with chronic fatigue syndrome are high achievers—people who want to get the most out of their life. People who have dreams and desires. CFS does not affect lazy people.

It is really important for family members to understand that CFS doesn't play fair. Its name doesn't reflect its crippling truth. It robs you of your life. It robs you of joy.

Let's say there is a young woman called Jenny; an elite sports player. Jenny was always bubbly and popular at school. Until suddenly Jenny can't do what she used to be able to do. She's in bed. She's sick, sore, and she's got unruly symptoms like brain fog, fatigue, weak immune system, muscle aches, flu-like symptoms, swollen glands, dizziness, sensitivities, and deconditioning of the body. She can't be the Jenny that everyone knows her to be, so she suffers from stress, anxiety, worry, shame, guilt, depression, anger and frustration. She is stuck in a negative loop. It's painful and she is constantly worrying about her health and her future. Jenny is no longer the happy-go-lucky person she used to be because she can't be! She's sick and plagued by a bewildering illness that she can't see but feels every day of her life. She feels isolated and lost.

How would it feel if you were Jenny?

It's important for family members to know what happens with shame, guilt and worry. Because while CFS is not an emotional problem, the physical nature of it *creates* emotional issues. In short, you can't live the life you want to live. It causes an array of emotional pain which ignites even more physical symptoms. It's like being stuck in a vicious cycle that you can't control.

It's not just days that tiredness, brain fog, and other symptoms persist either. It is the months and months (and sometimes even years) of being sick. And the longer it goes on, the more emotionally taxing it is. Think about when you're on day 3 or 4 of the flu, or if you've ever had gastro, and you're ten hours in and you think, *This sucks, I just want to be better again.* All you want is your life back, right? Imagine that pain but tenfold, sometimes for months, years or even decades for some people.

One of the biggest things about chronic fatigue syndrome is the chronic guilt and the shame that people have in regard to their family. They desperately wish they could get better so that their mom, dad, or people around them don't have to see them suffering and care for them. It's a heavy burden to carry, and only adds to the stress of the illness.

It's hard to watch a loved one suffer. But it can change, and it can get better. It's important to realize that you're doing the best you can. It's not going to be perfect. You're going to have misunderstandings with people you love. You're going to feel angry and frustrated. But one key thing is to have open communication, share how you're actually feeling, and also put up healthy boundaries. In this chapter there are some really helpful guidelines for loved ones so they can support your recovery and everyone can all be on the same page.

IF YOU LACK A NETWORK

If you don't have the support you need from loved ones, then look outside of it. Consider getting a coach or mentor who might be able to help you, or find people who have gone through your experience and recovered.

Social media is great for utilizing connections from all around the world, and there are support groups online that you can join for free. We have one at CFS Health with thousands of members globally, and it's a safe space to get support from people who know what you're going through. It's refreshing and nourishing to be around people who "get it."

Getting support gives you the mental clarity to focus on being forward-thinking and proactive, not reactive. Even the simple act of someone saying "that happens to me too" can be so reassuring to hear. Finding your tribe can be a life-changing experience.

A CAREGIVING INSIGHT
From Elana (Mother of Carly)

My daughter Carly had chronic fatigue syndrome, and my friends and extended family simply didn't understand what was happening to her. People would say to me, "Well, why doesn't your daughter just go and lie down and go to sleep and then she'll be okay?" I think the fact the illness is called chronic fatigue syndrome trivializes what it really is, and people didn't get it. They didn't understand that it's not just physical, it's also a full-blown mental and physical shutdown.

I had no one to talk to, and chronic fatigue became me. I lived and breathed it from the moment I woke up to the moment I went to bed. And it got to a point where I could feel that I was going into this black hole because I was obsessed with it 24/7, and it was affecting every aspect of me and my daily functioning. And that's when I realized I needed to go and see a professional and talk about what I'm feeling, even though I wasn't the actual one suffering from CFS, my daughter was, but it was affecting me. I needed to speak to someone neutral, who wasn't going to just give advice but simply understand.

Going to see a professional created a safe space. It wasn't a judgmental space, and it allowed me to be honest and express what I was feeling - my sadness and my own suffering. I was taking so much on board that I was like a pressure cooker.

I think it's important to seek outside help, not within your own circle, and especially not to the person suffering. They don't need that right now. You need to take time out for yourself, whether it's 15 minutes to one hour or even more, but literally set a boundary and don't stop doing things that are good for you.

At the end of the day, all you want is your loved one to be happy and healthy. It can be so hard watching from the sidelines wanting to help so much but at the same time you can't click your fingers and make them better. Recovery doesn't work like that.

As a carer, you should not feel guilty about enjoying your life. It's imperative that you find joy in your own day to day life which is going to give you energy. You need to make sure that you have hobbies, that you have things outside of the world of chronic fatigue syndrome to escape in a healthy way. This will stop you getting pent-up with frustration, anger and even resentment. Find ways that are healthy to express how you're feeling, but also express yourself through avenues of hobbies. For me, it's walking in the forest and playing piano. Whatever it is, find those activities that can get some separation from your "carer" identity to help you move forwards.

The other thing I would say is that you also need to make sure you get good sleep and adequate nutrition. There's a reason they say on airplanes to put your own oxygen mask on first— the healthier and happier you are, the better you will be able to take care of the person with CFS. You need the energy and boost to your wellbeing it provides.

You will also need to set boundaries, both for your relationship with the person you're caring for but also for your own health. You can be an emotional sounding board, but having boundaries will ensure it isn't exhausting for you too. You might have one hour a day where the person can tell you everything that is on their mind and you just listen and be supportive. At this time, it can be helpful to ask them if they want support or solutions—our first instinct when someone tells us a problem is to race to find a solution, but sometimes people want to vent and get their thoughts out even though they may already know the solution or find it themselves.

I also learned that when I was overzealous with my daughter's progress, it wasn't actually helping her. I would go, "Oh my God, that's amazing. I'm so excited." By saying things like this, I was putting pressure on her and making the situation about me and my excitement for her. Instead, I learned to say, "I'm pleased for you." To me, saying this means I'm not putting added pressure or placing my expectation that there will be continual progression each day. It doesn't quite work like that.

Letting go of the micromanaging of your loved one is a process. In the beginning, that's what you have to do to survive and we're part of that journey of helping them survive. But as the person recovers, we also must learn to start letting go, even if we have these fears and anxieties. We have to learn how to let go of that micromanaging so we are not projecting our concerns and fears onto them, and we can engage in life too.

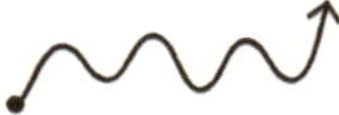

DOS AND DON'TS FOR CARERS

Don't Try to Cure the Person You Are Caring For

The person you're caring for doesn't need any more pressure than what they already place on themselves. I'm sure you have good intentions, but those good intentions can be misinterpreted as pressure. A common one is, "Come on, you can do this. You're going to get there."

When someone's feeling so low and flat, overly positive sentiments are the last thing they want to hear. They can be interpreted as pressure to get better faster. Recovery has to come from within, and everyone's on a different journey.

Try to avoid phrases like:

"Come on, you can do it."

"Push yourself just a little bit more."

"Think more positively."

In fact, it can do more harm than good. I once worked with a young lady whose father was a famous sports star in Australia.

When they first started the recovery program, I could sense the pressure from her father. He just wanted her better so she could get on with her life. Because of his work ethic and high status as a sports star, he expected the same level of commitment from his daughter. But the "working harder" or "pushing yourself" mentality doesn't work for CFS recovery.

Four sessions in, the young lady seemed a bit upset. I asked her if she was okay.

She replied. "Not really, Dad keeps telling me I need to push myself more, that I need to be more motivated and that I am just too lazy. I feel so much pressure it's horrible."

Then and there I knew I had to have a hard conversation with her father for the benefit of his daughter's health.

The call went something like this.

"Hey, it's Toby Morrison from CFS Health. Your daughter is in my recovery program and I wanted to call you to share some things with you. Firstly your daughter is on the right track; even though progress won't be huge right away, she's setting up her foundation, stopping the push-crash cycle and she will be able to start slowly progressing soon. The key is not pushing her beyond her limits or putting any unnecessary pressure on her. I know this may be hard to hear as a famous sports player who thrives on pushing hard and staying motivated all the time. But CFS requires the opposite initially.

I know this is hard and I know you're saying everything out of love and good intentions for your daughter, but I need you to stop telling her that she needs to be more motivated and push herself more.

Her recovery is her recovery, not yours. Be the supportive father that you are, but let her run her own race, you need to trust her process and allow her to learn and grow at her own pace."

Now of course it was a pretty awkward conversation to have with a man that probably isn't used to being told what to do, but it was the right thing for his daughter's health and recovery.

That lovely young lady started progressing really well over the following months, her and her dad developed a deeper and more beautiful relationship where he stopped trying to make her better but instead just loved her and supported her for where she was at. A year later they were able to go on an overseas surf trip together. She is now recovered, works full time, and travels the world, chasing waves for fun!

Just remember that chronic fatigue syndrome is enough pressure, they really don't need more pressure on top of what they already have.

Don't Over Celebrate Their Wins

Recovery isn't a linear process, so this is why it's important not to over celebrate their wins. You can absolutely be happy and proud of them for making progress, but by going overboard, it can make them feel guilty or like a failure if that progress dips back down the next day or the following week. When your loved one is doing a bit better and is more functional around the house and building up their capacity, you want to work as a team. Understand their current capacity and have a more relaxed approach. Instead of celebrating their progress as a concrete milestone (e.g., emphasizing how happy you are that they can now walk with you to the shops everyday), take things day by day (e.g., say "I'm proud of you for walking to the shops today" and don't put any pressure or expectations for them to do the exact same thing tomorrow or next week). This gives them the flexibility to listen to their bodies rather than push themselves to meet your expectations, even if they were given accidentally.

Try to avoid over-the-top style cheerleading (no pom-poms and high kicks required). At the end of the day, you know your loved one best and so taking some time to think of a balanced approach with encouragement that will be most beneficial for the person with CFS can be really useful.

I know that this advice is a bit tricky—you don't want to downplay their wins either, but I have seen a tendency for loved ones to go overboard with enthusiasm and it can be counterproductive. I totally understand how exciting progress can be...it's hard not to scream with joy when your loved one has a little 'win' but try to be chill if you can. Match their level of excitement, don't exceed it.

Don't Overshare or Be Super Emotional

Cry and express your emotions, but not in front of them. I've had lots of parents through the CFS Health program who have sought professional help to express their emotions to a neutral party in a healthy and meaningful way. Crying or expressing your frustrations or sadness in front of the person is not going to help them. You can of course do so in a way that lets them know you care, and you are empathetic toward them, but crying in front of them all the time or showing big expressions of sadness and other emotions only adds to the pressure and guilt they already feel about trying to get better. They're dealing with a life-changing illness already, they don't need to carry the guilt that they're changing your life too.

Don't Ask Them How They Are Feeling Too Much

I recommend you have a conversation with your loved one and say, "I want to let you know that I care about you a lot and I'm here to help you, but I also don't want to overwhelm you by asking how you are every one hour or three hours. So how about we have a deal that I'll ask you less and if you are stuck or you need help, you tell me and I'll be there."

I'm sure your loved one would be appreciative of that. You've got to stop checking in all the time, as it's not helpful and it can make the person feel suffocated or like they need to relive their symptoms every time they tell you. But I also get that you need to show them you care (it wouldn't be nice if someone never asked you how you were), so it requires forming a balanced approach that will be beneficial to you and the person.

I had to tell my dad to stop when he was doing the same thing. He would ask me constantly "Are you okay? Are you okay?"

I finally said, "Dad, I need you to stop asking me if I am okay all the time, it doesn't make me feel good." We had a massive conversation, and I said, "If I need help, I'll come to you. But other than that, we're good."

It was a game-changer because I didn't focus on how bad I was feeling all the time. And when we don't focus on how bad we're feeling, we start to focus on the things that we can do. And when we focus on the things we can do, we can move forward.

Don't Expect Them to Be the Same Person They Used to Be
It can be both beautiful and challenging to witness your loved one's recovery. As they heal, they may rediscover parts of themselves that were long suppressed by illness—new interests, boundaries, or a renewed sense of purpose. This transformation can sometimes feel like you're getting to know a different person. It's important to remember that growth often brings change, and while it may take time to adjust, this evolution reflects a life no longer defined by illness. It's important to minimize expectations about them "returning back to their former self" and allow them the freedom to simply be who they are now.

Do Let Go of the Micromanaging
There comes a time to let go of micromanaging. As they recover, they will regain their agency and it's important to let them have

it. They will know what is right for them, so let them be the judge and be in control. They will start to be more functional, cooking for themselves and doing chores. They will probably enjoy this! Your first instinct might be to tamper them down so they don't go backwards in their recovery, but you have to trust they know what they are doing and allow them to take their recovery into their own hands.

Over time, you're going to let them grow and slowly take a step back. You can still provide encouragement and support, but it could be a matter of having a conversation and saying, "You're doing really well. If you need me, I'm here for you, and if you don't, then that's good too." That way you can get on with your normal life and they can move forward.

Do Stop Researching and Suggesting Solutions All the Time

When your loved one gets sick, it's totally natural to do a heap of research and provide solutions. You're like, "Oh, why don't you try this?" or "I've researched this stuff, maybe you should try that." While this can be good in moderation, doing too much is very overwhelming for the person and can put pressure on them to try everything that's out there rather than focusing on the pathway they've actually chosen to take.

I once had a client who was the son of a very well-known wealthy man from Europe. He was a pretty intimidating guy and he called me one night and he said, "He's not getting better. He needs to push himself more." I knew the approach he had taken with his son's recovery and I had to have a hard conversation then and say, "You need to stop pushing him and stop telling him how he needs to live his life. The more you do that, the longer this is going to go on." He took my advice on board, He started to get better, and after six months, he was a different person. At the time, he thought he was doing all the right things and throwing money at all these pills and supplements, but it was actually hindering the recovery process because he was putting massive expectations of recovery onto his son.

When the person is bombarded with solution after solution, it only creates pressure to heal and do everything that their loved ones want them to do. It also creates this sense of anger because people often offer solutions that won't actually do anything but they think they're gifting you the secret. What you need to remember is that they are in control of their health and they need space to have that agency.

There will come a time when you'll be able to let go of the caregiving reigns, and go back to simply being their loved one.

Do Remember the Bigger Picture

When one person in the family is sick, it can be easy for life to begin revolving entirely around them. This is natural in the short term, but over time it's vital to protect the fabric of family life. You can do this by keeping up family routines, events or rituals, even if they need to be scaled down or made appropriate to the person's capacity. For instance, if the family goes to the cinema every Saturday night, rather than forgoing it altogether, you could have a special movie night at home with popcorn and snacks and make it as close to the cinema experience as possible. This keeps the fun and spirit of the ritual without it getting lost by not going. The idea is to make it special.

It also creates a space that does not revolve around the person's illness and helps them to focus on the family and the ritual. You can also help the person take their mind off their recovery by creating space for joy, humor, hobbies, and normalcy—these are healing too, but without the pressure of working toward a goal that is directly linked to recovery.

Recovery is a journey and so is learning how to love and support someone through it. Boundaries, honesty, and shared moments beyond illness can make that path smoother for everyone involved.

Do Let Them Learn Lessons

Supporting someone through chronic fatigue syndrome can be an emotional balancing act. One of the more challenging dynamics can be when your loved one becomes hyper-focused on their recovery. While their intention is valid—healing takes focus after all—it can sometimes result in overwhelm, both for them and for those around them. This is where setting healthy boundaries and creating emotional structure comes into play. Sometimes you can't force lessons. Letting the individual make mistakes and learn from them is part of the healing process.

Do Let Go of the Perception of Your Loved One Being Ill

This is a very, very big one. One of the most powerful shifts you can make in supporting someone with CFS is letting go of the constant perception of them as "ill." Yes, they are managing a complex and often invisible condition—but if your focus is always on what they *can't* do, it will be harder for both of you to see what they can. Your perception becomes part of their reality. If you treat them as fragile, they may start believing they are.

Letting go of the "illness identity" doesn't mean denying what they're going through—it means choosing to see and affirm their wholeness, strength and progress. It's seeing them not only for their symptoms or illness, but for the full human being they are.

Doing this will support their self-belief, as when you see them as resilient rather than ill, it reinforces their ability to trust their own body and mind again. It will also change the energy between you—conversations and interactions become lighter, more empowering, and less about what's wrong—and it invites progress. People are more likely to stretch themselves and step forward when they don't feel boxed in by other people's expectations.

How to Let Go

Avoid over-accommodating

Ask what they want help with instead of assuming what they need and listen to what they say. If they say they don't need help, then don't give it anyway just because you think they need it.

Focus on shared moments, not symptoms

Bring in more connection points outside of their illness—games, conversations, rituals you both enjoy.

Avoid making adaptations they didn't ask for

Sometimes making adaptations for someone who is ill, while absolutely thoughtful, can make them feel embarrassed or dehumanized. An example is if you automatically brought a chair over for them to sit down every time they enter a room, without checking if they need it. While the intention is caring, it can unintentionally send the message that you see them as weak or incapable. These kinds of unsolicited gestures, though well-meaning, can undermine their autonomy and reinforce an identity of illness they may be trying to move beyond. Just ask them if they need help.

Let them be the boss

If you're doing an activity, let them make the decision on what they're capable of doing. You can offer a specific alternative rather than making the choice for them. For instance, if you're on a walk and one path goes uphill while another one stays flat, you can simply ask, "Should we go the flat route today?" rather than saying, "Let's go the flat route for you" or "You can't go uphill, so let's go the flat way."

This mental and emotional shift is subtle but profound. When you focus on their strength instead of their suffering, you give them one of the greatest gifts: the belief that recovery is not only possible—it's already in motion.

THE 3 PHASES OF SUPPORT

There are three common phases that occur during recovery. The carer's role within these three phases often changes according to the sufferer's stage of recovery. Let's walk through them together and I will offer some practical tips and tools for helping your loved one *and* yourself too.

Phase 1—the acute phase.

This acute phase is when the person is at 1, 2 or 3 out of 10 in terms of their energy levels. They are usually suffering very much—physically, mentally, and emotionally.

For the sufferer—during this phase, you want to decrease the amount of physical and mental stress as much as you possibly can. From household chores, cooking, cleaning, moving things, and general daily tasks. The body is in a high state of stress trying to recover, so decreasing stress here is key.

For the loved one/carer—during this phase your physical output is quite high so it is vital that you look after yourself too.

DO:

- Help with the physical basic needs.
- Get outside help, such as cooking or cleaning.
- Be an emotional sounding board but have your own boundaries.
- Speak in an open, honest way with kindness.

- Seek help for YOU.
- Talk to someone outside the relationship, such as a coach or a psychologist, (not family or friends).
- Take time out for yourself each day.
- Look after yourself with good sleep, good nutrition, and movement that you enjoy.

DON'T:
- Be over-eager to help with every single thing.
- Be overly positive or try to motivate them.
- Use phrases like: "Come on, you can do this," or "push yourself," or "think more positively."
- Overshare or be emotional in front of a loved one. Cry but not in front of them. Express your emotions away from the loved one.
- Over celebrate their wins.
- Don't get too involved, good or bad. Stay neutral.

Phase 2—the reconditioning stage

The reconditioning phase is when your loved one is doing a bit better, they're more functional around the house and building up capacity. They are usually between a 3-6 out of 10 in terms of energy levels. This is where you want to work as a team.

Understand their current capacity and also have a more relaxed approach.

You will let go of the micro-managing and instead they will take a more active role in their recovery.

They will still need to rest and stay within what feels appropriate for them. It isn't uncommon that they can start to cook for themselves, do basic chores (even enjoying it) and start to become more functional in everyday life.

For the sufferer—it's a great time for conversation; such as discussions around current boundaries and new boundaries.

For the loved one/carer—your loved one still needs you to support them but you'll find it will be a bit more relaxed and include conversations around non-recovery topics. During this stage, you will need to navigate and explore their new needs (as well as your own) and decide what feels appropriate. It's important to still be considerate and kind but also allow them to grow into their own level of progress.

For the loved one/carer:

DO:
- Keep encouraging them.
- Allow their process and stay in your own lane.
- Allow them to take some responsibility but ensure it feels appropriate.
- Connect about things outside of recovery.
- Let go and allow their experience.
- Keep living your life and care for them when you need to (but you'll find it won't be intense like the acute phase).

DON'T:

- Push them or say "Come on, hurry up."
- Place expectations on them.
- Be over-controlling.

Phase 3—the integration stage.

The integration phase is when your loved one is between a 6-10 out of 10 in terms of daily function. They are ready to integrate back into life.

With this phase comes a lot of challenges. Don't be surprised if your loved one begins to feel stressed; it's a part of integrating back into life. Entering back into 'real life' is not always easy and this is why we have an uplevel program called Lifestyle Integration 2.0—it's designed to support members as they recover and enter back into the big wide world.

For loved ones—just continue to love and support them and allow them to have their own learnings and understandings. The conversations often change from recovery challenges to life challenges, which isn't a bad thing.

For the one in recovery—you no longer have as many recovery challenges, so now it's life challenges. What to do with more energy and more time? What work/career/study/hobbies do I choose?

When a person with chronic fatigue syndrome is in phase 3 and reintegrating back into life, there are still some obvious dos and don'ts for the loved one.

DO:

- Keep encouraging them, but allow them to have their own process. You stay in your own lane.
- Allow them to take on some responsibility, but don't put responsibility on them that they didn't choose.
- Start re-engaging in the things you enjoy doing together, like cooking together, going to the movies, or going for a walk. Before chronic fatigue syndrome came along, you did things together and enjoyed each other's company, so it's important to prioritize that again.

DON'T:

- Stay stuck in the perception of them as ill but instead see them as healthy.
- Remain in a state of being overprotective, it's not helping at this stage.
- Re-live recovery conversations or experiences that no longer serve them.

The role of the caregiver is always driven by love: the will to want your loved one to feel empowered again, to be in control of their life again; to feel joy and energy and happiness again. And this goal should also be the same for you too.

TAKEAWAYS

<hr>

NAVIGATING RELATIONSHIPS: It is often as hard for a loved one to see you suffer as it is for you to go through it. I remember how upset my mom was. She told me she wished she could change bodies with me. I also know how hard it is sometimes for some family members to fully understand what's going on with you. Sometimes it can cause a lot of tension and there's a lack of understanding, knowledge and support around this entire topic.

IF YOU LACK A NETWORK: If you don't have the support you need from loved ones, then look outside of it. Consider getting a coach or mentor who might be able to help you or find people who have gone through your experience and recovered. When you get support, it gives you the mental clarity to focus on being forward-thinking and proactive, not reactive.

UNDERSTANDING CFS: Chronic fatigue syndrome isn't in the mind. It's a very real neurological and physical illness. It's a full shutdown of the body and people often have eight or more symptoms persist for a period of six months before getting diagnosed, and they are not only dealing with the physical symptoms, but also a whole lot of emotional chaos from essentially losing their previous life.

DOS AND DON'TS FOR CARERS: While there are a few main things you can do to protect your relationship with the person with CFS and provide essential support, the main things are to approach the situation with understanding and empathy and to not smother them with attention and solutions, instead prioritizing their agency and control over their health.

LETTING GO OF THE "ILLNESS IDENTITY": One of the most powerful shifts you can make in supporting someone with CFS is letting go of the constant perception of them as "ill." Yes, they are managing a complex and often invisible condition—but if your focus is always on what they *can't* do, it will be harder for both of you to see what they can. Letting go of the "illness identity" doesn't mean denying what they're going through—it means choosing to see and affirm their wholeness, strength and progress.

WHAT TO DO WITH HYPER-FIXATION: One of the more challenging dynamics can be when your loved one becomes hyper-focused on their recovery. While their intention is valid—healing takes focus after all—it can sometimes result in overwhelm, both for them and for those around them. This is where the art of setting healthy boundaries and creating emotional structure comes into play. Have a conversation about setting times for discussions around their recovery and prioritize protecting as much of the family rituals as possible.

RECOVERING INSPIRATION

Carers and loved ones can watch this documentary together and see some real stories of real families getting better.

CHAPTER 13

THE RECOVERY COURAGE LEAP

To think recovery is a walk in the park is like saying to a young kid that it's easy to ride a bike first with no training wheels. It's hard and there will be lots of ups and downs and times when you feel like giving up. It takes a lot of courage to reach the stage of acceptance and move forward with your journey, and even more courage to keep on going when things feel hard or scary.

Recovery is hard but *not* recovering is harder.

It takes courage to heal. To try a new way of being. To reach for hope without any guarantees. But we must lean into courage and not shy away from it. We must get comfortable with being uncomfortable and forge a new way forward. This doesn't mean we get to remain unscathed, because that's not possible. But we do get to emerge stronger and wiser and with more love and compassion. As the great Khalil Gibran wrote, "Out of suffering have emerged the strongest souls; the most massive characters are seared with scars."

Every new level of recovery and healing invites a new level of expansion within you. I have always said that going through chronic fatigue syndrome is a spiritual journey. Not in a woo-woo kind of way, but in the life-changing sense. You will not emerge as the same person who went in. Yes it hurts, yes it's hard, but on the other side of recovery is a meaningful life, one you haven't even imagined before. You become a more evolved person—a person who has found meaning, a person with purpose and gratitude. There is a depth you gain from going through something like CFS.

Here are some real-time displays of courage that are required during recovery.

- Letting go of the idea that there is a quick fix solution = courage
- Accepting where you are at so you can start to change it = courage
- Letting go of your old identity so you can rebuild a new one = courage
- Letting go of friendships and relationships that no longer serve you in your recovery = courage
- Letting go of guilt = courage
- Choosing yourself = courage

- Fully dedicating yourself to yourself and your future = courage
- Not chasing shiny objects and going down quick fix rabbit holes = courage (and commitment)
- Staying true to yourself = courage
- Progressing and going to new levels (outside of your comfort zone) = courage
- Pure dedication and focus on the right things = courage
- Saying no = courage
- Saying yes to the hell yeses = courage
- Believing in yourself even when there are doubts = courage
- Staying the course, even when progress is slow or non-existent initially = courage
- Not giving up, even though you feel like it = courage
- Being honest with yourself = courage
- Acting on your dreams and aspirations = courage

As you can see, recovering from chronic fatigue syndrome requires courage. A tremendous amount of courage. And this is why recovery isn't easy. A lot of people confuse confidence with a feeling of ease and happiness. Yet confidence is courage, commitment, plus doubt.

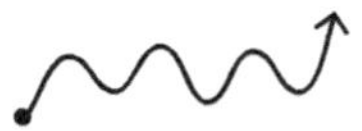

~~~~~~

**It won't always feel easy and that is okay.
Every new level requires a new
level of expansion within you.**

~~~~~~

What got you here, will not get you there—and so it is up to you to expand to new levels—physically, emotionally, cognitively, and spiritually.

As I said at the start of this chapter, going through chronic fatigue syndrome *is* a spiritual journey. Not in a woo woo sense, but in a life-changing sense. Yes it hurts, yes it's hard, but on the other side of recovery, is a meaningful life, one you haven't imagined before.

Today, choose courage.

Whenever you feel like you're not doing enough or you've hit a setback, I want you to list all the ways you have shown resilience and courage in your journey.

Ways I showed resilience and courage in my journey:

____

____

____

____

____

KRISTI'S RECOVERY

Kristi is a mother of two from the USA. Before becoming sick, Kristi was very active. She was a public school teacher who went on to homeschool her own children. While homeschooling, they traveled to over 140 national parks, monuments and sites. Started two La Leche League groups and trained leaders for breastfeeding moms in Stockton, volunteered with a prison ministry, started a hiking Meetup; organized and led over 300 hikes, sat on a few various boards, coached soccer and swimming, was a missionary in Mexico, trained as a bowen therapist and lactation counselor, and was an athlete. She had swum the Escape from Alcatraz race, hiked the John Muir Trail, and was working her way through hiking/climbing the 14,000+ ft mountains in California. People considered Kristi a Type-A personality and she was extremely empathetic and wanted to help others as much as possible. She was a self-prescribed people pleaser, and often felt she wasn't doing enough.

Kristi had symptoms on and off for over a decade but numerous tests showed nothing. Her symptoms got worse (swollen lymph nodes, heart palpitations, twitching eye, "vomit days" where she couldn't move or she would vomit). She could barely function. Kristi became bed and homebound. She couldn't take a handful of steps without collapsing. She could not digest solid foods for a month. The pain grew so intense that she would curl up in the fetal position, grab her head, and wish death would come.

She said, "I felt like my organs were shutting down. I needed to be in a dark, quiet room and no longer could read or communicate more than a few sentences with my teenage children, husband, family or a few special friends. Some days were better and I could move to a sofa with sunglasses on. Rarely did I leave the house. Curling up into a ball on the cement walkway, floor of an elevator, or within the door of a doctor's office would normally be very embarrassing and "dramatic," but there came a point where I just didn't care. Not because I wanted attention (please don't see me weak), but because I just didn't have the energy to care.

My family moved out of a valley and onto a mountain. We thought I would die within the year, so we were willing to try the move. I was able to be seen and diagnosed by Stanford's Chronic Fatigue and Infectious Disease Clinic, as well as a homeopath in my home town. There was very little hope as my homeopath told me I would never hike again, and my Stanford doctor asked if I needed his help getting on disability. It was a dark, painful time.

Upon joining CFS Health I found hope, validation, and guidance. Hope is the foundation of recovering. Having a community of hundreds of like minded people rooting each other on is huge! Joining CFS Health was the kickstart I needed for recovery to happen.

The love, guidance, support, accountability, and accessibility was great for me."

Kristi can now eat most foods without any issue. She no longer needs to wear sunglasses inside, Her memory of words and conversations has returned and the brain fog has lifted. She can move, drive, dance and run without PEM. She still gets normal tired when she overdoes things but knows how to create healthy boundaries. She is not only hiking, after recovery, but she is climbing, kayaking and paddleboarding. She is able to mountaineer again, and finished the list of 14K+ ft. peaks in California. They traveled as a family to Mexico, South Africa, Italy, Montenegro and Greece to celebrate her son and daughter's high school graduations.

Kristi says, "I try to live a balanced life as much as possible. I have learned to enjoy just being, but I am living and "being" at the same time now. Being is living too. I am loving myself wherever I am. I am loving life."

How cool is Kristi's story. And there are so many similar ones like hers.

If you want to hear Kristi's full inspiring story, check this out:

ACKNOWLEDGING YOUR RECOVERY

I believe with the right support, everyone will get their recovery story.

When we post success stories and interviews, there's usually always one person who posts a comment like, "they're just one of the lucky ones." It actually makes me angry seeing those types of comments because it is disrespectful to the person who has usually dedicated years getting their life back. I have watched them overcome so many hurdles, do the work, and continue to grow and expand from their recovery over many months. There's no such thing as luck, they did the right things at the right time, consistently, to get the right results.

It's important to recognize the work you do, even when no one sees how hard you are trying or suffering; the silent moments of faith and the inner traits that helped you along the way.

Let's acknowledge them and write them here.

I am most proud of my:

____

____

____

____

Resilience	Dedication	Compassion
Strength	Belief	Never give-up
Courage	Humor	attitude
Tenacity	Trying	
Kindness	Caring nature	

The Courage You Need, You Have

It takes a quiet, persistent kind of courage to recover from chronic fatigue syndrome. Or any chronic illness for that matter. It's not the kind of courage that gets headlines or medals (although recovering from CFS does deserve a medal)—it's deeper (and harder) than that. It's the quiet strength to try. It's the choice to believe in healing, even on the days when your body is screaming at you.

Recovery from chronic fatigue syndrome isn't always a straight line. It's not a victory you get to shout from the summit of a mountaintop one grand day. It's about reclaiming your life, step by step. It's in the decision to keep going when progress is invisible. It's in the patience you give yourself on the hard days, and the grace you offer when your limits grind to a halt and your body says, "no more."

Courage is saying *"I will keep showing up for myself"*—not because it's easy, but because your life is worth it. Because you are worth it.

No matter how long the road has been, or how many times you've been knocked down and had to start over, you are *not* weak—you are incredibly strong. It takes more strength than people would know to keep saying yes to your life, to keep putting one foot in front of another when all you want to do is give up.

I see you. I see your courage. I see your worth. Find the message in the mess, be open to change and possibility. I have seen too many people who once thought they were never going to get better actually overcome this condition and go on to living their lives again. Recovery is possible.

Recovery doesn't have to be forever, but health is. Focus on recovery now, so one day you can just focus on being healthy and living your life again.

Toby Morrison

CONNECT WITH US

If you are looking for more help and support with your recovery, here are 4 ways CFS Health can help you.

 Download our free recovery trainings at www.cfshealth.com

 Watch our life-changing documentary—
Freedom - Healing from Chronic Fatigue Syndrome
www.cfshealth.com/freedom

 Listen or watch our Chronic Illness Recovery Podcast episodes on YouTube, Spotify or Apple.

YOUTUBE   SPOTIFY

 **Join our Online Recovery Program**
Get a comprehensive recovery plan with coaching, accountability, and community support that helps you with every step of your recovery so you can get healthy and start living again: www.cfshealth.com/form

For more information about getting your life back, email info@cfshealth.com or visit www.cfshealth.com

ACKNOWLEDGMENTS

Thank you to Amanda Cooper and John Morrison for being incredible parents, and to my sister, Johanna Morrison, for being my go-to source of unwavering support during hard times. You have all been my light in the darkness. Your support and encouragement have been unwavering throughout my life, and I will never forget everything you did to help me get better.

A special mention to Dr. Lubitz for being the first doctor to believe in me and to tell me that recovery was possible, even though there was no pill to cure it.

A huge thank-you to my entire team at CFS Health—many of whom were once clients recovering from chronic fatigue syndrome. Your enthusiasm and commitment to helping people from all around the world get their lives back give me purpose.

A special mention to Ash Ward, the general manager at CFS Health, for going through the book one last time to make sure every word counted and added value to the reader's life. No pages were left unturned. Thank you for your patience and for helping me bring this book to life.

Thank you to John Marsh for encouraging me to add more stories to this book to show the real truth of recovery and the inspiring legacy the work at CFS Health has created.

Thank you to the team at Dean Publishing, particularly Natalie Deane, who worked with me to make sure this book was clear, practical, and, most importantly, easy to read. Thank you for your work and dedication to my mission.

ABOUT THE AUTHOR

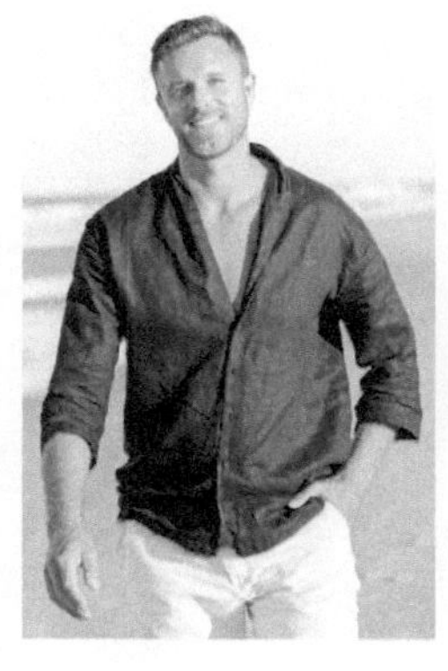

Toby Morrison is the founder of CFS Health, which was created in 2009 as Australia's first health center solely dedicated to helping people with chronic fatigue syndrome. CFS Health established the first "done-with-you" Recovery Program, which has been online since 2013 and continues to run today, helping thousands of people in more than seventy-eight countries.

CFS Health stands for Choice, Freedom, and Success, which is what Toby has created for himself and thousands of others.

Toby founded CFS Health after enduring a long and frustrating journey to recovery. At the age of sixteen, he became ill with chronic fatigue syndrome and suffered for four years. Recognizing the lack of awareness and effective, practical treatments, Toby and his team of health professionals developed a safe and effective online recovery treatment program and community.

Toby also published his first book, *Chronic Fatigue Syndrome: A Guide to Recovery*, in 2013.

The recovery processes Toby and his team have developed have also helped people with ME/CFS, fibromyalgia, POTS, post-viral fatigue, and long COVID. If you have been diagnosed with any of these conditions, the models and frameworks from CFS Health will show you a proven pathway to restore your health and start living again.

www.cfshealth.com

AUDIOBOOK

Get Your Life Back is also available in audio format.

Jump onto your favorite audiobook platform
to have the story narrated for you by the author.

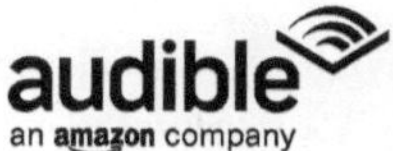
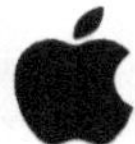
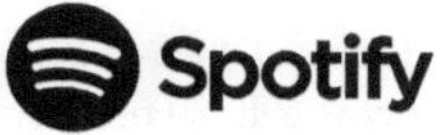

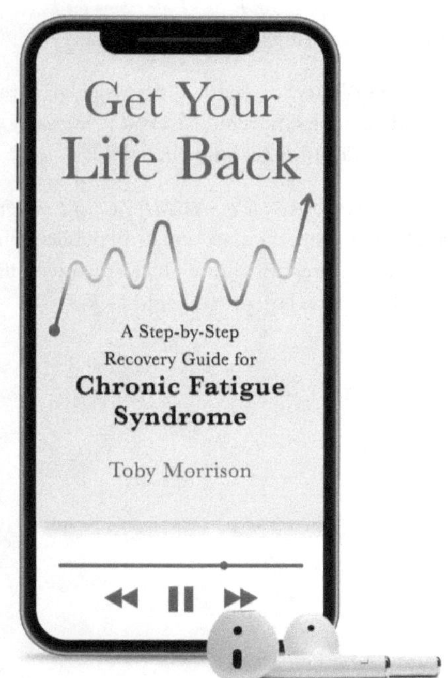

ENDNOTES

1   Zhou, Yuting, Yating Zhang, Chenyi Liu, and Wenyan Zhang. 2023. "The Effect of Nutrition and Health Education on Patients with Chronic Fatigue Syndrome: A Randomized Controlled Trial." *Evidence-Based Complementary and Alternative Medicine* 11 (2). https://doi.org/10.3390/healthcare11020223

2   Sapra, Armit, and Priyanka Bhandari. 2023. *Chronic Fatigue Syndrome*. Treasure Island, FL: StatPearls Publishing.

3   Better Health, "Immune System Chronic Fatigue Syndrome", (n.d) https://www.betterhealth.vic.gov.au/health/conditionsandtreatments/chronic-fatigue-syndrome-cfs

4   White, K P et al. "Co-existence of chronic fatigue syndrome with fibromyalgia syndrome in the general population. A controlled study." *Scandinavian journal of rheumatology* vol. 29,1 (2000): 44-51. doi:10.1080/030097400750001798

5   Lipton, B. H. (2005). *The Biology of Belief: Unleashing the power of consciousness, matter and miracles*. Mountain of Love/Elite Books.

6   Fulcher, K Y, and P D White. "Strength and physiological response to exercise in patients with chronic fatigue syndrome." *Journal of neurology, neurosurgery, and psychiatry* vol. 69,3 (2000): 302-7. doi:10.1136/jnnp.69.3.302

7   *ME/CFS Advisory Committee Report to the NHMRC Chief Executive Officer*, 2019https://www.nhmrc.gov.au/about-us/publications/mecfs-advisory-committee-report-nhmrc-chief-executive-office r#block-views-block-file-attachments-content-block-1